Critical Thinking *in* Long-Term Care Nursing

Skills to Assess, Analyze, and Act

SHELLEY COHEN, RN, BS, CEN

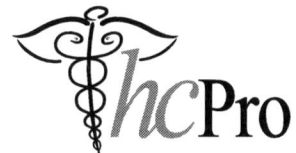

Critical Thinking in Long-Term Care Nursing: Skills to Assess, Analyze, and Act
by Shelley Cohen, RN, BS, CEN, is published by HCPro, Inc.

Copyright © 2008 HCPro, Inc.

All rights reserved. Printed in the United States of America.   5 4 3 2 1

ISBN 978-1-60146-137-7

No part of this publication may be reproduced, in any form or by any means, without prior written consent of HCPro, Inc., or the Copyright Clearance Center (978/750-8400). Please notify us immediately if you have received an unauthorized copy.

HCPro, Inc., provides information resources for the healthcare industry.

HCPro, Inc., is not affiliated in any way with The Joint Commission, which owns the JCAHO and Joint Commission trademarks.

Shelley Cohen, RN, BS, CEN, Author
Polly Gerber Zimmerman, RN, MS, MBA, CEN, Contributing Author
Janie Krechting, BSN, RN-C, MGS, LNHA, Contributing Author
Noelle Shough, Editor
Emily Sheahan, Group Publisher
Janell Lukac, Graphic Artist
Michael Roberto, Layout Artist
Susan Darbyshire, Art Director
Sada Preisch, Proofreader
Darren Kelly, Books Production Supervisor
Susan Darbyshire, Art Director
Claire Cloutier, Production Manager
Jean St. Pierre, Director of Operations

Advice given is general. Readers should consult professional counsel for specific legal, ethical, or clinical questions.

Arrangements can be made for quantity discounts. For more information, contact:

HCPro, Inc.
P.O. Box 1168
Marblehead, MA 01945
Telephone: 800/650-6787 or 781/639-1872
Fax: 781/639-2982
E-mail: *customerservice@hcpro.com*

Visit HCPro at its World Wide Web sites:
www.hcpro.com and ***www.hcmarketplace.com***

1/2008
21349

Contents

List of figures vi

About the authors viii

Introduction: Critical thinking in the long-term care setting x
    Back to basics x
    Critical thinking and the long-term care setting xi
    Assessment xii
    Treatment and management of resident care xiv
    Discharge and implications to long-term outcomes xvi
    Encouraging the development of critical thinking in long-term care nurses xviii

Chapter 1: Defining critical thinking 1
    Why critical thinking? 1
    Becoming a professional nurse 1
    So what is critical thinking? 2

Chapter 2: New graduate nurses and critical thinking 7
    Why don't new graduates think critically? 7
    New graduates' levels of development 10
    Prioritization 10
    Identifying worst-case scenarios, stereotypes, and expected abnormal findings 13
    Ongoing development 15

Contents

Chapter 3: The critical-thinking classroom 17
    Critical thinking can be taught 17
    Background preparation 17
    Setting the stage 19
    Classroom content 21
    Classroom processes 27
    Instructional approach and style 28

Chapter 4: Orientation: Bringing critical thinking to the clinical environment 49
    Moving from the classroom to the bedside 49
    Beginning with orientation 51
    The role of preceptors 54
    Teachable moments 57
    Handling judgment or action errors during orientation 61
    Orientation sets critical-thinking expectations 64

Chapter 5: Nursing practice that promotes and motivates critical thinking 67
    Maintaining momentum 67
    Nurse managers and staff educators 68
    Making critical thinking part of the culture 70

Chapter 6: Novice to expert: Setting realistic expectations for critical thinking 77
    Setting realistic expectations 77
    Novice to competent: New graduate nurses 78
    Greatest challenges for new graduate nurses 79
    Competent to expert: Experienced nurses 82
    Measuring critical thinking in daily practice 84

Chapter 7: Applying critical thinking to nursing documentation 87
    Turning critical thinking into critical writing 87
    Examples of critical writing skills for long-term care nursing 91

Chapter 8: Relating critical thinking to its higher purpose 97

Chapter 9: Resources and tools 99
    Resources and further reading 99
    Additional sample questions.. 103

List of figures

Chapter 3

Figure 3.1: Teaching Critical thinking—Critical-thinking course content and prioritization handout 31

Figure 3.2: Teaching critical-thinking skills—Sample course content, objectives, and scenarios 42

Figure 3.3: Teaching critical-thinking skills—Classroom tips 44

Figure 3.4: Teaching critical-thinking skills—Sample self-assessment tool 46

Figure 3.5: Teaching critical-thinking skills—Handout 47

Chapter 4

Figure 4.1: Critical-thinking self-assessment tool—General nursing skills 50

Figure 4.2: Critical-thinking self-assessment tool—Long-term care nursing skills 52

Figure 4.3: Preceptor tool—Relating skills to critical thinking for new graduate nurses 56

Figure 4.4: Preceptor tool—Relating resident observations to critical thinking 58

Figure 4.5: Preceptor tool—Promote and support critical thinking 59

Figure 4.6: Successful orientation requires critical thinking 65

Chapter 5

Figure 5.1: Critical-thinking skills assessment—Nurse manager/staff educator tool 69

Figure 5.2: Annual performance review—Self-assessment of critical thinking 73

Figure 5.3: Goals worksheet 75

Figure 5.4: Setting goals for improvement 76

List of figures

Chapter 7
Figure 7.1: Eight common charting errors 88

Chapter 9
Figure 9.1: Critical thinking skills course—Additional resources handout 109

Figure 9.2: Unfolding teaching scenarios for long-term care nurses 112

Figure 9.3: Skilled unit teachable moments 117

Figure 9.4: Critical-thinking skills and the frail elderly in the nursing home setting 120

Figure 9.5: Sample agenda 122

Figure 9.6: Instructor worksheet—Connecting words to spark critical thinking 123

Figure 9.7: Nurse worksheet—Connecting words to spark critical thinking 124

Figure 9.8: Worksheet—Relationship to critical thinking 125

Figure 9.9: Worksheet—Vital signs 126

Figure 9.10: Worksheet—Red-flag alerts 127

Figure 9.11: Worksheet—Relating nursing care to critical thinking 128

About the authors

Shelley Cohen, RN, BS, CEN

Shelley Cohen, RN, BS, CEN, is the founder and president of Health Resources Unlimited, a Tennessee-based healthcare education and consulting company (*www.hru.net*). Through her seminars for nursing professionals, Cohen coaches and educates healthcare workers and leaders across the country to provide the very best in patient care. She frequently presents her work on leadership and triage at national conferences.

When she is not speaking or teaching, Cohen works as a staff emergency department nurse and develops educational plans for a local emergency department, including strategies for new-graduate orientation. She also writes her monthly electronic publications—*Manager Tip of the Month and Triage Tip of the Month*—read by thousands of professionals across the United States.

She is an editorial advisor for **Strategies for Nurse Managers,** published by HCPro, Inc., and is a frequent contributor to *Nursing Management* magazine. She is the author of *Critical Thinking in the Emergency Department, Critical Thinking in the Obstetrics Unit, Critical Thinking in the Pediatric Unit*, and coauthor of the book *A Practical Guide to Recruitment and Retention: Skills for Nurse Managers*, all published by HCPro, Inc.

She has a background in emergency, critical care, and occupational medicine. Over the past 30 years, she has worked both as a staff nurse and nurse executive.

When her laptop computer shuts down and her stethoscope comes off, Cohen puts on her child-advocacy hat and, with the help of her husband, Dennis, provides foster care to area children.

Contributing author: Polly Gerber Zimmermann, RN, MS, MBA, CEN

Polly Gerber Zimmermann, RN, MS, MBA, CEN, has been active in emergency and medical-surgical nursing clinical practice for more than 29 years and involved in nurse education for more than 10 years. She was the senior course manager for the nursing division of the National Center for Advanced Medical Education, and is a tenured assistant professor in the Department of Nursing at the Harry S. Truman College (Chicago). Under her guidance, the school's curriculum instituted an integration of prioritization principles and critical thinking that resulted in the school's students improving from below to above national average results in these areas on standardized test scores.

Zimmermann is a frequent national speaker and has published more than 200 times. In addition, she writes test items that score high in critical thinking for national standardized tests, including HESI, NLN, NCLEX, and Excelsior College (Regents).

She was an associate editor and section editor of the Managers Forum for the *Journal of Emergency Nursing* for more than 10 years and is a contributing editor for the emergency section of the *American Journal of Nursing*. She has also been a legal expert/consultant in more than 45 cases.

Contributing author: Janie Krechting, BSN, RN-C, MGS, LNHA

Janie Krechting, BSN, RN-C, MGS, LNHA, is a clinical consultant and assistant professor of Aging Services and Administration at the College of Mount St. Joseph in Cincinnati. She is also the author of the books *Clinically Based Long-Term Care Survey Preparation Guide Manual*, *Interdisciplinary Care Plans for Long-Term Care*, and the *Quick Guide to Documentation*.

Krechting's consulting expertise is on OBRA compliance, PPS/RUGS III, MDS/RAI, quality improvement, assessment, documentation, care planning, management, and supervision.

Introduction: Critical thinking in the long-term care setting

By Janie Krechting, BSN, RN-C, MGS, LNHA

LEARNING OBJECTIVES

After reading this section, the participant should be able to:
- Describe the characteristics of the long-term care setting that require good critical-thinking skills

Back to basics

The complexity of care and increasing resident acuity seen in the long-term care setting today require critical-thinking skills beyond those required even just five years ago. Since the inception of the hospital diagnosis-related groups (DRGs), nursing home residents resemble the medical-surgical patient from pre-DRG days.

As nursing schools respond to the shortage of nurses by increasing enrollments, decreasing the length of time it takes to become a nurse, and thus increasing the output of new graduates, nursing homes are seeing a greater need for graduates to display critical-thinking skills and strong mentors to help nurses develop those skills.

In contrast to reality, there is public sentiment that long-term care nurses are inferior in knowledge and skill to hospital nurses. The long-term care nurse actually must be just as sharp as, if not sharper than, acute care nurses because the long-term care nurse must be an extension for the physician. Physicians are only required to see residents every 30 days in the long-term care setting, in contrast to the daily visits required in the hospital.

This creates the need for the long-term care nurse to be a strong critical thinker and a strong mentor for new nurses entering the profession. This book provides some skills, tools, and tips

Introduction

to assist nurses as they hone this process to make it as natural as breathing. The fundamental concepts of critical thinking are essential for long-term care nurses because they must meet the challenges of being a new nurse and being compliant in the most heavily regulated industry in the United States.

To make the most of this book as your resource for critical thinking, consider taking time to review all of the content before you implement the helpful tools. It may be tempting to just start using the tools immediately, but resist. It sounds strange that you should not immediately use the tools provided, but just as you would not expect a new nurse to understand the relationship between blood loss and delay in blood pressure changes without some foundational knowledge of anatomy and physiology, you too will not be able to fully understand the implications of the tools provided without doing some critical thinking of your own. The tools are not the answer: The answer lies in grasping the concepts of critical thinking.

Critical thinking and the long-term care setting

Depending on where you work, there can be a constant stream of chaos as residents move into and out of the unit, or the unit can be a relative island of calm. Sometimes it can be both on the same day. Nursing home units can vary from a subacute unit housing residents with high-acuity needs, including ventilator services, suctioning, wound care, and intravenous therapy, to a rehabilitation unit, an Alzheimer's unit, a hospice unit, or a generalized floor.

The unknowns that make long-term care such an interesting place include:
- How many residents have risk factors, such as high risk for pressure ulcers?
- How many residents will be high acuity or low acuity?
- How many residents have the potential for behaviors?
- How many have the potential for delirium or confusion and are therefore a risk to themselves?

Geriatric nurses stand alone much of the time as they deal with the issues presented by their particular patient load. The sense of teamwork seen in hospital departments, such as the emergency room or the operating room, is often not as strong in the long-term care setting. In part, this is due to the high turnover rate, as nurses move from nursing home to nursing home, but

Introduction

it is also the nature of the work being done. Long-term care nurses care for a wide variety of residents and need to apply knowledge of a wide variety of conditions and risk factors. For this reason, the need for extraordinary critical-thinking skills is imperative.

Nursing homes are as different as they are numerous—there are more than three times as many nursing homes as there are hospitals. A nursing home may be focused on a specific type of resident (e.g., rehab or Alzheimer's) or it may be a mixed unit that takes all types of residents regardless of the illness or management of a chronic disease and its implications on long-term care. This broad variety ensures two things: first, that the long-term care nurse will never be bored, and second, that the need for critical thinking is essential as the nurse deals with multiple demands.

The three main areas in which the long-term care nurse will need to apply critical thinking are assessment, treatment, and management of resident care, and discharge and implications to long-term outcomes.

Assessment

Whether residents present as direct admits from the hospital, home, or another facility, a sorting process occurs to determine their potential for injury to themselves or others through delirium or other cognitive needs, their potential for demise, or the need to keep them close to the nursing station for easy access to extra assistance. This area of nursing practice requires not only critical thinking, but also experience, and it is usually managed by the nurse manager or the unit shift leader/charge nurse.

Once a resident is physically placed in the unit, the charge nurse must also determine the skills needed by the nurse who will care for this resident as well as the current workload of the nursing staff. The most successful unit shift leaders/charge nurses are those who possess an ability to think critically about multiple factors, the implications of those factors, and their use when making effective decisions. Clearly, this is not a process new-graduate nurses are prepared for without extensive experience and learning opportunities. But new graduates will be expected to care for these residents once they are placed in the long-term care unit. That too creates a need for critical thinking in even the least experienced nurses as they determine and meet the needs of the residents they receive.

Attributes of critical thinking during resident care

The following examples demonstrate application of the concepts and approaches of critical thinking at the point of care in the medical-surgical unit. Strategies and attributes of critical thinking during care include the following abilities:

Independent thinker

- Analyzes and initiates the written orders as presented with the resident.
- Recognizes when workload associated with resident volume will require more support and notifies nurse manager/charge nurse.
- Reconciles medications ordered with those that the resident is known to be taking and ensures that all are accounted for or ordered if necessary.

Evaluates evidence and facts

- The report from the emergency room nurse states that the resident fell down a flight of stairs and broke her hip and arm. At initial assessment when the resident arrived on the unit, the nurse notes a number of large bruises that are in various stages of resolving. The resident lives with a caregiver who is presently staying very close to the resident.

Explores consequences before making decisions or taking action

- A multiple sclerosis resident's dad takes her to the store, but staff report that the resident's mom, who has had a severe cardiovascular accident and is unable to communicate, was left in the resident's room unattended while the dad and the resident are gone.

Evaluates policy

- Recognizes that although a visitor is demanding to see the resident now, the resident's chart indicates there is a restraining order against the ex-husband. The charge nurse is contacted prior to allowing any visitors through the door.

Confident in decisions

- On admission the resident reports that she feels nauseated. Rather than beginning an immediate assessment, including a mobility assessment, the nurse decides to administer an ordered antiemetic and allow the resident to settle in before the full assessment is done.

Introduction

Asks pertinent questions

- Understands that no assumptions should be made on admission. Every resident is assessed from head to toe and is asked pertinent questions regarding areas of skin breakdown, poor nutritional status, living conditions, or domestic abuse.
- Asks when the resident last had a bowel movement.

Displays curiosity

- At admission, begins to look at the picture of the resident's reported living conditions and starts to think about what will be needed in order for the resident to go home when he or she is ready to leave.

Rejects incorrect information

- Notes that although the caregiver states that the resident has been taking all of his cardiac medications, the resident has +3 edema to the lower extremities and cardiac arrhythmias that would normally be controlled by the medications.

Treatment and management of resident care

There have been many changes in the long-term care setting over the last few years that have resulted in a rapid turnover of residents. Residents used to stay in the hospital for many days as their long-term treatment plans were resolved. Now residents are often shifted to a rehabilitation or skilled nursing facility for finalization of their care, potential transfer to long-term care, or return to the home environment.

Long-term care facilities vary, but they offer the opportunity for critical thinking. Physicians, residents, and families are all more dependent on the assessment and critical-thinking skills of the nurse than in a hospital setting. In an environment that faces rapid staff turnover, and where 12 hour-shifts are not uncommon, the skill to assess change of condition and when and what to do about it is essential.

Attributes of critical thinking during treatment

Strategies and attributes of critical thinking during the treatment process include the following abilities:

Independent thinker

- Identifies and rationalizes which residents need prioritized attention.
- Recognizes the need to call pharmacy to ensure two medications are compatible.

Evaluates evidence and facts

- Notes critical lab values, reassesses resident, and approaches provider with information and request for orders.

Explores consequences before making decisions or taking action

- A resident who had a knee replacement surgery done three weeks ago has been less mobile than the physical therapist and the provider would like. The resident is to be discharged to home tomorrow and has been in bed all day today except for bathroom visits. The resident is taking anticoagulant therapy and has requested a day of rest before going home tomorrow.

Evaluates policy

- Resident is unable to care for herself and has new bruises of unknown origin. Nurse refers to facility policy requiring all suspected abuse situations be reported.

Confident in decisions

- A provider challenges the nurse about contacting him at 3 a.m. about a change in a resident's condition. The nurse is able to refer the provider to the specific changes in vital signs and the subsequent discussions with the unit shift leader/charge nurse that triggered the call. The challenge should be communicated through the chain of command so that the medical director can work with the team, review policy, and assure nurses that they may call 24 hours a day without fear of reprisal from the physician.
- During a resuscitative effort, a physician orders a dose of medication that is twice the dose recommended by the American Heart Association. Despite the urgent needs of the resident, the nurse reads the order back to the physician and questions the dose.

Introduction

Asks pertinent questions

- The nurse is comfortable saying, "This resident's vital signs are stable but there is something that we have not identified yet that is concerning me. How do you feel about my doing an EKG on her?"

Displays curiosity

- When caring for a chronic pain resident, the nurse approaches the provider and, while updating him or her on the resident's status, inquires, "Do you know anything about chronic pain residents being given anti-Parkinson's medications in addition to their usual dose of narcotics? This resident is demonstrating tolerance of his narcotics and we have tried almost all of the narcotics available. Do you think this might work for this resident?"

Rejects incorrect information

- When reviewing laboratory results in the computer, notes a resident has dangerously low blood sugar. After reevaluating the resident, the nurse performs a finger-stick glucose test and finds the resident to have normal-range blood sugar. Upon discussion with the lab, it is determined there is another resident with the same first and last name of this resident on another unit.

Discharge and implications to long-term outcomes

After the planned treatment has been provided and the resident is ready for discharge, the options for where a resident goes next include:

- Discharged home
- Returned/admitted to another nursing home as resident
- Transferred to another facility for further care (e.g., a Veterans Administration Medical Center)
- Sent to the morgue

With more residents waiting for an empty bed, there is always a push to move residents out of the unit as efficiently as possible. The added pressure of moving residents in and out of the unit quickly is an additional obstacle for nurses trying to employ critical thinking. As part of the discharge process, nurses need to consider the following:

Introduction

- Nurses must reevaluate vital signs, pain status, neurological status
- Nurses must review documentation to ensure completeness and thoroughness
- Residents with limited English proficiency take longer to discharge
- Some discharge instructions are lengthy or complicated
- It may take time to await the appropriate person, other than resident, to review discharge information
- Discharges being held until someone can come to pick them up require ongoing nursing assessments

As mentioned before, the nurse must also consider the home situation of residents and whether or not they have the physical ability to manage stairs and care for themselves once home. Does the nurse manager, Minimum Data Set coordinator, or social worker need to be involved in the resident's discharge? The expectation is that the nurse will consider all of the aspects of care needed for safe management after the resident leaves the facility. It is important that nurses have the time and resources they need to accomplish everything with critical thinking and critical documenting.

Attributes of critical thinking during discharge

Strategies and attributes of critical thinking during the discharge process include the following:

Independent thinker

- Recognizes the discharge orders from the provider are premature and the resident will need to wait for an evaluation by the mental health worker, social worker, or nurse manager.

Evaluates evidence and facts

- Although resident claims, "I can handle this by myself," nurse notes resident is unable to demonstrate safe use of a walker. Suggests to provider that the resident be seen by physical therapy for a further assessment before discharge.

Explores consequences before making decision or taking action

- Asks who will be driving the resident home prior to administering a narcotic for pain management.

Introduction

Confident in decisions
- Although a particular dressing is ordered for the resident's pressure ulcer, the nurse recognizes the fragile skin of the resident and suggests another option that will not require tape on the resident's skin.

Asks pertinent questions
- Asks elderly resident who lives alone, "Is there someone who can help you with these dressing changes when you get home?"

Displays curiosity
- When discussing the resident's functional status, determines if there is a specific cause for the functional decline.

Listens to others and is able to give feedback
- Requests a return demonstration from a resident admitted for therapy and newly diagnosed insulin-dependent diabetes mellitus. The resident is going home alone.

Encouraging the development of critical thinking in long-term care nurses

Much of the critical thinking needed in the long-term care setting comes from work experiences with other nurses and in dealing with particular resident scenarios. Nurses tend to remember specific situations and the cascade of events that occurred to create a particular outcome. It is the shared knowledge of all nurses that can provide the best mentorship to new-graduate nurses. Sharing that learned experience with other nurses can increase the critical thinking abilities of peers and provide excellent learning experiences for others.

For this reason, all nurses should be actively involved in the orientation and development of both new-graduate nurses and experienced nurses who join the unit. Without passing along these clearly remembered cascades, we cannot help others to develop their critical-thinking capabilities.

We want long-term care nurses who are able to:

- Recognize a problem
- Know what to do
- Know when to do it
- Know how to do it
- Know why they are doing it

Long-term care nurses know what outcomes they want for each resident and recognize how they personally and collectively affect those outcomes. Recognizing the role critical thinking plays in achieving these desired outcomes is the first step to creating and achieving an environment that promotes sound judgments.

It is a privilege to be a long-term care nurse and be at the side of a resident and family when they are in need of medical care. It takes a special person and comes with a tremendous responsibility and power to make the best decisions with and for the residents who have entrusted their care to us.

Chapter 1
Defining critical thinking

By Polly Gerber Zimmermann, RN, MS, MBA, CEN

LEARNING OBJECTIVES

After reading this section, the participant should be able to:
- Identify key aspects of critical thinking
- Explain how nurses develop competency in critical thinking

Why critical thinking?

For educators and nurse leaders, critical thinking is like the weather: Everybody is talking about it, but nobody seems to know what to do about it. Passing the NCLEX only validates that new graduates have the minimal amount of knowledge needed to provide safe nursing care. Application of clinical critical thinking and judgment is at the heart of what makes a healthcare provider nurse (as a verb) compared to being a technician who completes tasks by rote. Critical thinking is at the core of safe nursing practice, and thus encouraging its development in every nurse should be an aim for all educators.

Becoming a professional nurse

Nursing is a hands-on profession for which clinical experience plays a crucial role in professional development. Nurses have to progress through various levels before they reach proficiency. Managers and educators need to appreciate that new graduate nurses are at a different level, with different needs, than experienced nurses in their professional critical thinking.

Benner's stages of growth

Benner (1984) is well known for identifying and describing the five stages through which nurses proceed in their professional growth.

Chapter 1

> **Benner's stages of growth**
>
> **Beginner:** Has little experience and skills. Learns by rote, completing education requirements.
>
> **Advanced beginner:** Can perform adequately with some judgment. Nurses are usually at this stage upon graduation.
>
> **Competent:** Is able to foresee long-range goals and is mastering skills. Still lacks the experience to make instantaneous decisions based on intuition. Most nurses take up to one year to reach this stage.
>
> **Proficient:** Views situation as a whole, rather than its parts. Is able to develop a solution.
>
> **Expert:** Intuition and decision-making are instantaneous. Most nurses take at least five years in an area of practice to reach this stage.

So how do you take your inexperienced graduates and set them on the road to proficiency? And how do you help your more experienced nurses—who may have been practicing for years, yet you would never label them experts—reach that higher level? This book provides information, strategies, and tools to help you coach nurses at all stages of development as they hone their critical-thinking skills, improve their judgment, and become better nurses. Chapter 3 discusses teaching critical thinking in a classroom setting, and other chapters include ongoing strategies for developing critical thinking in the clinical environment.

The goal in encouraging and developing critical thinking is to help nurses progress effectively through the stages of development. No one wants 10-year nurse employees who have the equivalent of one year of experience simply repeated 10 times.

So what is critical thinking?

Alfaro-LeFevre (1999) defines critical thinking as careful, deliberate, outcome-focused (results-oriented) thinking that is mastered for a context. Critical thinking is based on scientific method; the nursing process; a high level of knowledge, skills, and experience; professional standards;

a positive attitude toward learning; and a code of ethics. It includes elements of constant reevaluation, self-correction, and continual striving for improvement.

Some of the characteristics of people who display critical thinking include open-mindedness, the ability to see things from more than one perspective, awareness of one's own strengths and weaknesses, and ongoing striving for improvement. The strategies commonly (and often subconsciously) used in critical thinking include reasoning (inductive reasoning, such as specific to general, or deductive reasoning, such as general to specific), pattern recognition, repetitive hypothesizing, mental representation, and intuition.

In the practical world of clinical nursing, critical thinking is the ability of nurses to see patients' needs uniquely and respond appropriately, beyond or in spite of the orders. The ability to think critically is developed through ongoing knowledge gathering, experience, reading the literature, and continuous quality improvement by reviewing one's own resident charts. An example of a nurse who displays critical thinking is when a physician orders acetaminophen (Tylenol) for a resident's fever, and the nurse questions the order because the resident has hepatitis C. A critical thinker goes beyond being a "robo-nurse" who simply does as he or she is told.

In Croskerry's study (2003), 32 types of misperceptions and biases (cognitive disposition to respond) were identified in clinical decision-making. Everyone is influenced by what they see most often, most recently, or most dramatically. Cognitive errors may be avoided by always striving to consider alternatives; by decreasing reliance on memory (instead, use cognitive aids such as reference books); by using cognitive forcing strategies, such as a protocol; by taking time to think; and by having rapid and reliable feedback and follow-up to avoid repeating errors.

The overarching goal is to help shorten new graduate nurses' on-the-job learning curve, and give directed assistance to all nurses in their critical-thinking development.

Del Bueno's definition of critical thinking

There are many definitions of critical thinking, and one of the most helpful is Dorothy Del Bueno's Performance-Based Development System. Del Bueno determined that nursing competency involves three skills: interpersonal skills, technical skills, and critical thinking.

Chapter 1

Del Bueno defines critical thinking in a clinical setting with the following four aspects:

- Can the nurse recognize the resident's problem?
- Can the nurse safely and effectively manage the problem?
- Does the nurse have a relative sense of urgency?
- Does the nurse do the right thing for the right reason?

Let's use a scenario to solidify the point. Say a resident becomes more confused than usual, and demonstrates verbally aggressive behavior. The expectation is that nurses will recognize that this could potentially be related to a urinary tract infection, rather than assuming it is appropriate to immediately order an antipsychotic. In addition, the nurse will know to complete a dipstick to assess the resident for other signs and symptoms of urinary tract infection, such as fever, burning on urination, etc. The nurse will know to encourage fluids, especially cranberry juice, obtain a specimen, contact the lab to collect the specimen, and then notify the physician when results arrive.

Overall, Del Bueno found that nurses' greatest limitations were in recognition and management of renal and neurological problems. Inexperienced nurses may only focus on the resident's behavior.

REFERENCES

Alfaro-LeFevre, R. 1999. *Critical Thinking in Nursing: A Practical Approach.* Philadelphia: WB Saunders.

Benner, P. 1984. *From Novice to Expert.* Menlo Park, CA: Addison-Wesley.

Brown, S. 2000. "Shock of the new." *Nursing Times* 96 (38): 27.

Charnley, E. 1999. "Occupational stress in the newly qualified staff nurse." *Nursing Standard* 13 (29): 32–37.

Croskerry, P. 2003. "The importance of cognitive errors in diagnosis and strategies to minimize them." *Academy of Medicine* 78 (8): 775–780.

Del Bueno, D. 2001. "Buyer beware: The cost of competence." *Nursing Economics* 19 (6): 257–259.

Gries, M. 2000. "Don't leave grads lost at sea." *Nursing Spectrum.* Accessed on July 27, 2006, from http://community.nursingspectrum.com/MagazineArticles/article.cfm?AID=800.

Huber, D. 2000. *Leadership and Nursing Care Management,* 2nd ed. Philadelphia: WB Saunders.

Norris, T. L. 2005. "Making the transition from student to professional nurse." In B. Cherry and S. R. Jacob, *Contemporary Nursing: Issues, Trends, & Management,* 3rd ed. St. Louis: Elsevier/Mosby.

Tingle, C. A. 2000. "Workplace advocacy as a transition tool." *LSNA Insider* (June).

Zimmermann, P. G. 2002. "Guiding principles at triage: Advice for new triage nurses." *Journal of Emergency Nursing* 28 (1): 24–33.

Zimmermann, P. G., and R. D. Herr. 2006. *Triage Nursing Secrets.* St. Louis: Elsevier/Mosby.

Chapter 2
New graduate nurses and critical thinking

By Polly Gerber Zimmermann, RN, MS, MBA, CEN

LEARNING OBJECTIVES

After reading this section, the participant should be able to:
- Analyze the factors that contribute to new graduates' lack of critical thinking
- Identify strategies to facilitate critical thinking in new graduates

Why don't new graduates think critically?

Educators' and nurse leaders' desire to develop nurses' critical thinking is undoubtedly more pressing for new graduate nurses. You may wonder why these nurses, who have just completed their education, do not display the qualities and skills you either expect or want. It's important to understand that new graduates face many stresses as they transition from students to registered nurses, and these stresses impede their ability to learn and progress.

Stresses for new graduate nurses

Charnley (1999) identified four categories that lead to stress in novice nurses.

Chapter 2

> **Stresses for new graduate nurses**
>
> 1. **Reality of practice:** They think they are supposed to have all the answers, are overwhelmed by the volume of work, and feel guilty because they cannot spend more time with residents.
>
> 2. **Unfamiliarity with the structure of the organization:** They spend valuable time looking for supplies.
>
> 3. **Lack of professional relationships:** They lack an understanding of the roles of healthcare providers, and their dependence on other staff may cause anxiety. They often lack mentors and support people.
>
> 4. **Lack of clinical judgment:** They have decreased confidence in their skills and decision-making abilities. This leads to apprehension.
>
> Other special needs of new graduates have been identified, including the following (Brown, 2000; Charnley, 1999; Gries, 2000; Huber, 2000; Tingle, 2000):
>
> **Interpersonal skills/communication:** They struggle with interactions with other providers in making rounds, clarifying orders, and during interdisciplinary team conferences. They may miss some communication or instruction from an experienced nurse because they don't understand what the routine or slang involves. For example, a new graduate may not understand the NCS, or "No concentrated sweets," diet. The graduate may have only learned about an 800-calorie diabetic diet, which is rarely used in nursing homes.
>
> **Clinical:** Though new nurses possess the clinical knowledge, they lack the experience that increases effectiveness, efficiency, and correctness.
>
> **Organization:** This includes organization of skills and the day, often exacerbated by nurses feeling overwhelmed and unsure how to prioritize.

> ### Stresses for new graduate nurses (cont.)
>
> **Delegation:** New nurses often feel uncomfortable delegating to more experienced and/or older assistants. This is exacerbated by a lack of leadership skills and trust/personal knowledge of the assistants.
>
> **Priority setting:** Initially, there is a tendency to focus on tasks, rather than critical-thinking planning. This tendency extends to experienced nurses as well. It is a central issue in the provision of care. Charge nurses in nursing homes tend to focus on getting "medications passed."
>
> **Assertiveness:** There can be hesitancy to say no or to understand the difference between being assertive and being aggressive.

As outlined above, the transition into practice includes a lot of stress. But new graduates can be helped to overcome the stressors and grow in critical thinking more easily when the orientation process recognizes and deals with these stresses.

Strategies to minimize stress

There are aspects you can add to orientation and for ongoing use that will minimize these stressors for new graduates. Possibilities include:

- Holding regular support group meetings with fellow orientees.

- Using a mentor or assigning a buddy (or sponsor) who builds a relationship and will follow the nurse for at least a year.

- Holding a treasure hunt for supplies or other departments during their first week of work. It will help their confidence if they know where the laboratory is located when someone stops them in the hall to ask.

- Holding a roundtable of the institution's staff nurses who have been out of school for two to five years, who can offer tips and support. (These nurses will be experienced enough to have learned, but not so experienced to have forgotten.)

- Spending a day rounding with a physician or nurse practitioner who frequently admits to the unit.

Chapter 2

- Emphasizing the importance of just "tell somebody" when something is abnormal, even if they do not know the cause or the solution. Alerting someone else will help new nurses learn. Make clear that waiting, assessing, and hoping is not a good solution.

New graduates' levels of development

When learning a new field, there are four classic stages through which the person proceeds:

- Unconsciously incompetent
- Consciously incompetent
- Consciously competent
- Unconsciously competent

The most dangerous situation is when nurses do not realize what they do not know. The best orientee is the one who realizes when to ask for help. Surprisingly, weaker students are frequently very confident, in part because they don't grasp how much there is to learn or the potential risks.

A contributing factor to this phenomenon is that newer nurses are often placed on the off shifts with other inexperienced nurses. This can limit their exposure to more-experienced nurses and lead to them not realizing their deficiencies since their coworkers have similar levels of knowledge and judgment.

Part of developing critical thinking and orientees' ongoing self-knowledge should include encouraging them to think about "In what areas do I still need to grow?" Keep the issue of critical thinking and anticipation of potential resident complications in the forefront.

Prioritization

Prioritization typically is one of the most difficult aspects for new nurses to learn. They know if something is "normal" or "not normal," but struggle to know how much importance to attach to these classifications. Many educators and managers think new graduates will automatically pick up this discernment, but this often does not happen until after considerable time, exposure, and experience.

New graduates struggle to prioritize the needs within one resident, within a team of residents, and/or between resident and administration needs. It is necessary to provide rules and principles they can use until they develop and internalize their own clinical judgment and instinct.

Prioritization principles: Assessment

Many of the following concepts may seem simplistic and obvious, but remember that experienced nurses often forget what they, as new graduates, didn't know. Discuss the following aspects in a critical-thinking class, and include them during orientation and throughout new graduates' initial development:

Review Maslow's Hierarchy of Needs and ABCD: While familiar content, many new graduates have not specifically identified that "D for disability" includes mental status/level of consciousness (LOC), neurological and motor function, and pain. Pain, while not a good thing, is not always the worst thing. Sometimes in an effort to overcompensate for the past when analgesia received inadequate attention, pain is given almost absolute priority in the nursing curriculum. Two common areas of weakness in new graduates are failure to ask all aspects of a pain assessment (PQRST) and failure to note the severity within the ABCD prioritization. Use examples where the type of pain and/or location, rather than severity, alerts the nurse to the problem, such as a substernal pressure that the resident rates as a 5. Use examples in which the severity matters: a significant shock (Circulation) takes priority over a mild wheezing (Breathing).

Onset (sudden over gradual): True sudden onset of symptoms can signal a catastrophic event. It is a true "sudden" onset if the resident can recall the exact time or activity when it began, and the maximum intensity is reached immediately (in less than one minute).

Actual over potential: A common error of new graduates is to focus on a "more important" potential future problem than what is currently going on. For instance, they assume the asthmatic resident who states he or she will stop his or her prednisone will take priority over someone who is currently experiencing low blood pressure. Emphasize first things first: Treat actual problems before preventing a future one.

Systemic over local (life before limb): Something that has a systemic implication, or involves multiple systems, is a priority. If no other access can be obtained, an IV is started in the leg to administer the medication to treat sepsis.

Chapter 2

Trends: A trend, as opposed to an isolated incident, could be an indication of something more serious. Trends include a steady progressive decline, minor symptoms that recur repeatedly or increase in severity, and/or symptoms that are associated with other definitive (especially systemic) changes.

Compared to the resident's normal: Recognition of the same significant symptoms ("This is like the last time I had congestive heart failure") or identification of a new distinction ("This is different from any other headache I've had before") is important. When the complaint is "ordinary," such as a headache, remember there must be a reason why the resident thought it was important enough to report. Always consider the caregivers' perception of changes in the resident,
as they know the person better than anyone.

For example, one resident was reassured by three nurses that her reported urinary incontinence was "typical" for the elderly. It took the fourth nurse to assess this symptom as a new onset, with urinary burning, and take the necessary actions to diagnose the resident's new urinary tract infection.

Patient demographics: Certain groups are more vulnerable for rapid worsening or atypical symptoms and should receive more consideration. This includes the immunosuppressed, whether by age (the very young and the very old), medication (steroid administration), disease (diabetes mellitus, HIV/AIDS), or past history (splenectomy, donor organ recipient). Similarly, greater concern should be given to residents with multiple comorbidities (their systems are already taxed for coping and will be more easily overwhelmed), or a history of the "worst-case scenario" in the past for these symptoms (e.g., "This is just like I felt when I had my heart attack").

Prioritization principles: Time management

Medications tend to be a priority and new graduates should be encouraged to consider the type and timing of medications. Antidiabetic medications and antibiotics are usually given priority because of the consequences if they are not given in a timely manner. If two antibiotics are ordered for the same time, give the one with the shortest interval until the next dose first.

In school, nursing assessment and teaching are emphasized. The reality is that most hospitalized residents have a "diagnosis" and one of nursing's main functions is to properly administer the treatments prescribed for the resident's improvement. Why is the resident here? Make sure the "cures" are being administered.

Prioritization principles: Administrative

Residents before paperwork: Students from a heavily regulated industry, such as licensed practical nurses who worked in long-term care facilities, or those who truly understand legal implications, tend to overemphasize the documentation. Remind them that "post" charting is allowed if identified as such.

Stop any harm immediately: Those inexperienced in leadership tend to focus on others dealing with problems rather than directly taking care of it themselves. If an aide is making an error, go in and correct it now rather than telling the charge nurse, asking for more inservices, writing up an incident report, or even speaking to the aide at the end of the shift.

WHAT rather than WHO: An inexperienced nurse is likely to be intimidated and respond first to an authority figure who is barking orders. A serious resident need is always first. Have them role-play stating, "I must take care of this first, then I can be back and talk with you in about a minute."

Remind learners when talking about prioritization that everyone does receive care even if they are not first. Prioritization just recognizes that one person can only do so much at a time and there are competing demands. Prioritization involves the right care to the right person at the right time for the right reason.

Identifying worst-case scenarios, stereotypes, and expected abnormal findings

Worst-case scenarios

Another significant area in which new graduates need help is identifying and ruling out the worst-case scenario that could happen with a complaint. People make decisions heavily influenced by what they experience most often, most recently, or most dramatically in relation to the current situation. New graduates have mainly been exposed to textbook stable cases in clinical experiences.

Chapter 2

Give new graduates examples and specifically identify what would be the worst complication. Ask them how they would know the worst-case scenario was occurring when dealing with any resident, condition, or scenario. A long-term resident complaining of nausea may have the gastrointestinal flu, but has a fecal impaction been ruled out? How will the potential for constipation or impaction be assessed?

This is particularly important to stress during a critical-thinking class, but it should also be brought up again and again. Remember, repetition is the mother of all learning. New graduates should know that for each resident they take care of, they should first think, "What is the worst-case scenario?" so that this may be ruled out as necessary, and the process should eventually become automatic.

There is a familiar phrase used in medicine, "When you hear hoofbeats, think horses, not zebras." It illustrates the overarching principle that nurses should first consider the most common causes for a resident's presentation, but be alert to the fact that there are some "zebras" out there. Don't miss them.

Stereotypes

It can be helpful to include common misconceptions (which are often subconscious) in illustrations. For example, common stereotypes may include that psychiatric residents don't have physical problems, or that all old people are a little bit confused. Nurses should ascertain whether the elderly resident with new-onset confusion has low glucose, low pulse-oximeter reading, or a urinary tract infection. False assumptions can lead to a wrong action.

Expected abnormal findings

What is an expected finding for this given condition? Make the distinction that significant "abnormal" findings are not a concern when they are a part of that resident's known medical condition. It is not alarming that a resident with pneumonia receiving intravenous antibiotics has an elevated white blood cell count (WBC). It is more necessary to know if the WBC is higher, lower, or the same since starting the antibiotics.

It is not alarming that a resident with a diagnosis of diabetes mellitus has a blood sugar of 200, especially if the resident has a pattern of running high in the past. It is important to rule out complications such as changes in vision, skin integrity, or a fall related to dizziness.

Ongoing development

Awareness is the first step toward beginning to change behavior. Orientation often focuses on "how we do things here," and includes forms, policies, and the mission statement.

Orientation also should include a purposeful identification and focus on critical thinking. Discussion should include making clinical correlations, applying them to each resident's unique presentation, understanding the reason things are being done, and focusing on the most essential aspects in the proper order. Bringing these types of approaches to the forefront will help the new graduate understand what is needed to succeed.

REFERENCES

Alfaro-LeFevre, R. 1999. *Critical Thinking in Nursing: A Practical Approach.* Philadelphia: WB Saunders.

Benner, P. 1984. *From Novice to Expert.* Menlo Park, CA: Addison-Wesley.

Brown, S. 2000. "Shock of the new." *Nursing Times* 96 (38): 27.

Charnley, E. 1999. "Occupational stress in the newly qualified staff nurse." *Nursing Standard* 13 (29): 32–37.

Croskerry, P. 2003. "The importance of cognitive errors in diagnosis and strategies to minimize them." *Academy of Medicine* 78 (8): 775–780.

Del Bueno, D. 2001. "Buyer beware: The cost of competence." *Nursing Economics* 19 (6): 257–259.

Gries, M. 2000. "Don't leave grads lost at sea." *Nursing Spectrum.* Accessed on July 27, 2006, from *http://community.nursingspectrum.com/MagazineArticles/article.cfm?AID=800.*

Huber, D. 2000. *Leadership and Nursing Care Management*, 2nd ed. Philadelphia: WB Saunders.

Norris, T. L. 2005. "Making the transition from student to professional nurse." In B. Cherry and S. R. Jacob, *Contemporary Nursing: Issues, Trends, & Management*, 3rd ed. St. Louis: Elsevier/Mosby.

Tingle, C. A. 2000. "Workplace advocacy as a transition tool." *LSNA Insider* (June).

Zimmermann, P. G. 2002. "Guiding principles at triage: Advice for new triage nurses." *Journal of Emergency Nursing* 28 (1): 24–33.

Zimmermann, P. G. and R. D. Herr. 2006. *Triage Nursing Secrets.* St. Louis: Elsevier/Mosby.

Chapter 3
The critical-thinking classroom

By Polly Gerber Zimmermann, RN, MS, MBA, CEN

LEARNING OBJECTIVES

After reading this section, the participant should be able to:
- Determine classroom strategies to teach, promote, and support the development of critical thinking

Critical thinking can be taught

The tendency is to view critical thinking as an abstract formula to memorize. Rather, it is a process of applying acquired textbook knowledge to the clinical setting and specific residents. All nurses usually need some initial assistance in applying their knowledge to the situation, particularly for high-volume, high-risk, or infrequent resident presentations with which they have had little familiarity during their education or experience.

Classes that discuss and teach critical thinking can be beneficial for both new graduates and more experienced nurses. New graduates and new hires will benefit from classes held during orientation, but it also may be useful to periodically schedule general-attendance classes so that other nurses may participate.

Background preparation

Teacher preparation

Educators can tend to spend excessive energy on "what" to teach. Just as important is "how" to teach—determining the best way to communicate the information so learning takes place. When planning an educational session, focus less on "What am I going to say today?" and more on "What are my listeners going to learn today?"

Chapter 3

Teaching is not pouring wisdom into passive listeners. The teacher is a guide for active participation through a learning experience. Watch the audience's responses. That is the only way to perceive the need to repeat material, vary the presentation, or illustrate the content's application for this group.

Consider the learner's motivation

Why will attendees be motivated to learn? The driving force for all ordinary behavior is "What's in it for me?" Avoid the *Field of Dreams* approach—i.e., if we plan it, they will come and learn. Instead, use the human tendency toward selfishness—"What's in it for me?"—to teaching's advantage. Further breaking down that number-one motivation reveals the three main aspects people want from education sessions. People want to:

- Get something accomplished/meet their goals
- Receive personal recognition, power, or influence
- Have social interaction and enjoyment

Most of us are usually more influenced by one factor than another, but there are aspects of all three in everyone. Time spent in the classroom should meet all three purposes. Give certificates; have checklists to complete; give personal, positive, public praise; and add humor or games.

Generational differences

Understanding motivational aspects is important when considering today's multigenerational work force. Everyone is influenced by the time in which they were raised, when they developed their mindset, values, priorities, and styles. As the Arab proverb says, "People resemble their times more than they resemble their parents."

Baby Boomers are individuals born between 1946–1964. The average age for registered nurses is 44 to 47. Baby Boomers are more likely to act out of a sense of duty and a drive to accomplish.

Generation Xers are those born between 1965–1980. They want independence and flexibility; they want to know "Why?" (as they focus on results); and they want fun. If an activity is not worthwhile to them, they do not feel a sense of obligation to stick it out and will check out physically and/or mentally.

Generation Y is the generation born between 1981–2006. They are entering the workplace with high expectations for themselves, their employers, and their managers, and expect coaching, training, and support to help them achieve their goals.

Many educators fall into the Baby Boomer age category, whereas new graduate nurses often fall into the Generation X or Generation Y categories. Remember that approaches used for the established work force, or even for you when you were a new graduate, may not work now. It's important to tailor learning experiences to meet the needs of all generations in your classes.

Professional nurses' goals

David Shore (1997) defined what professionals want from their educational offerings: They want to be an ACE. Specifically, they expect Access (to peers, resources, and networking), Credentialing (external validation of what they know and whether it is still correct), and Education (information to make a demonstrable, practical difference in their practice).

Keep these expectations in mind when planning learning experiences. Also note that experienced nurses are very interested in regulations (e.g., "The Centers for Medicare & Medicaid Services requires . . . ") or legal requirements (e.g., "In this case, a nurse was sued for . . . ").

Setting the stage

Classroom environment

The classroom environment plays a key role in your critical-thinking course. Create an atmosphere that awakens the participant's whole brain and senses. Communicate, even on a subconscious level, that this is an enjoyable, desirable place and activity.

Chapter 3

Classroom environment

Seating: As much as possible, use a half-circle for small groups, and a fishbone configuration for larger groups. Avoid having a group at a table with stragglers in the row behind. Avoid hiders: Participation is necessary for learning.

Use color: One study found that visual aids with color and symbols increased long-term retention by 14–38%.

Peripheral learning: We use sight for 75% of our learning. While we speak at 125 words per minute, we think at about 600 words per minute. Give the learner something to do with the extra 475-word capacity. When their mind or eyes start to drift, let them fall on educational posters.

If it is a dedicated classroom, make posters that specifically apply to the content that is being taught. If it is a generic classroom, use prevention and healthcare associations' free posters—then even the housekeeping staff learns.

Music: Play upbeat music before class, during breaks, and after class. Baroque is recommended because it matches the rhythm of the heart and enhances learning. Use lively pop music with a distinct beat you can dance to—it will pump up the energy in the room.

Frequent breaks: Experts recommend taking a five-minute "exercise" break every 40–50 minutes, but it's even more effective to take a one-minute break every 25 minutes or so. Set a kitchen timer and, when it dings, announce that it's time for a break and turn on the music. Encourage general arm stretching, walking around, etc. Indicate participation is optional.

After one minute, turn off the music and start class, usually with a joke. These breaks should be in addition to the scheduled longer break midway through the class. Teachers fear these breaks will create a loss of control of the classroom but that does not happen with adults when done with purposeful actions and explanations. Many students indicate "the music break" was one of their favorite aspects of the class.

There are many reasons to take these frequent breaks. Necessary bathroom breaks are then quickly facilitated without disrupting the classroom—and those who straggle back in miss the reward of humor. Exercise increases cognitive functioning, attention, and alertness. It pulls in the kinesthetic learners and individuals who have minor attention-deficit problems.

However, the real purpose for the breaks is to aid learning. People remember the first and the last things—educators call this the primacy and recency effect. More breaks mean more "firsts" and "lasts" to make an impression on one's brain.

Classroom content

New-graduate content

When new graduates are asked about their biggest fears and concerns, they mention concerns about how to handle their many responsibilities (during school they only had to deal with one or two residents), how to handle emergencies (especially a "code"), and how to communicate with physicians/when to call the doctor.

The first step in teaching critical thinking may be to help them develop a plan of action to enable more effective responses when encountering these issues in practice. This will free up their energy to allow them to focus on the subtle resident care assessments and important interventions.

Use some of these tips as a starting point for discussion.

Getting work done

- Provide a cheat sheet form for taking report or for the day's organization.
- Set "drop dead" times within your day (such as "all 9 a.m. medications to be in the residents' bodies by 10 a.m.") as guideposts for your progress in the day's time management.

Chapter 3

- Work ahead. Always assume the unexpected will happen—it does.
- Keep current with your charting. It is harder to recall everything at the end of the day.
- Constantly reprioritize. Don't ask yourself, "What are all the things I should do?" but "What is most important for me to do?"

Emergencies/code

- Get help. For a code, if nothing else, go out in the hall and say, "I need help right now in room X!" in an urgent tone, with a loud, calm voice.
- Learn the facility's system for distinguishing a code from a "do not resuscitate" resident.

Contacting the physician

- Take the initiative and introduce yourself to the physicians who admit frequently to your unit.
- Rehearse introductory statements/scripts for common needs. "Your resident (name) in room X is reporting Y and requesting Z. Do you want to order anything at this time?"

General advice

- Be slow to join a clique.
- Make friends with the unit secretary.
- Make your rounds during the night whether others do or not.
- Make your own list of procedures or skills you have never experienced and let everyone on the unit (especially during orientation) know your desire to watch/participate in these tasks.

Teach in the context of clinical application

When planning a critical-thinking class for new graduates, experienced nurses, or both, remember that your session will be enhanced when the classroom time is spent applying knowledge to the clinical setting. Do not simply give a theory lecture. Instead, use images from books or sample labs.

For example, you could hold up a picture of a stage III pressure ulcer and ask, "What do you think you do when a resident is found with an area like this?" Or present lab results (see below) and ask which value nurses should take care of first.

Value	Result	Normals
Glucose	193 mg/dL	70–110 mg/dL
BUN	8 mg/dL	10–20 mg/dL
Cr	0.7 mg/dL	0.7–1.2 mg/dL
Sodium	131 mEq/dL	136–145 mEq/dL
Potassium	3.2 mEq/dL	3.5–5.0 mEq/dL
SGOT/ALT	1932 IU/L	13–40 IU/L
SGPT/AST	2360 IU/L	7–60 IU/L
Bilirubin total	2.9 mg/dL	0.2–1.2 mg/dL

Experienced nurses are likely to pick potassium, but new graduate nurses rarely do so. Nurses learn the importance of potassium levels in part from work experience. This exercise will shorten the learning curve. You can also ask additional questions, such as:

- What disease does the resident have?
- How does the resident look?
- Why isn't the sodium level the most important since it is "lower" than the potassium deficiency?

Prioritization

Nurses not only need to know what to do, but the importance and order in which things should be done. Nurses of all experience levels may need help with prioritization for multiple needs within one resident, between multiple residents, and between resident and administrative needs.

Chapter 3

> ## Case study
>
> **Prioritization doesn't always come naturally**
>
> At one associate-degree nursing program, the faculty had assumed students would naturally pick up the concepts of prioritization. The faculty was appalled when the students scored below the national average in this category on a standardized test.
>
> To remedy the problem, the nursing program added classroom time to talk about principles of prioritization, followed by a year-long integration of such principles into future content. By giving the problem a specific focus and emphasis, the school's students now score above national average in prioritization.
>
> The handout developed for the second-year students can be found at the end of this chapter (Figure 3.1). This tool can either be used during critical-thinking classes, or given to attendees as a take-home reminder.

Strategies to teach prioritization

One way to teach prioritization principles is to use sample test questions dealing with prioritization, followed by a discussion of the rationale. For example:

Question: It is most important for the nurse to care for which resident complaint first?

 a. Resident with type II diabetes mellitus with an a.m. blood sugar of 190 mg.

 b. Resident with a K+ of 3.2 mEq who is receiving a K+ rider IVPB and states his arm is sore.

 c. Resident reported to be having a seizure.

 d. Resident with pneumonia being treated with IV antibiotics for one day. Today's WBC is 14,000 mm3.

Answer:

The intended answer is C because a seizure represents an immediate crisis. Follow-up discussion could include the difference if A was hypoglycemic, normal side effects of potassium infusions, and the fact that D is already being treated. However, discussion should also include the need to look at trends. If this was the resident's third day on antibiotics and the WBC was the same or increasing, we would need to initiate action toward consideration of changing antibiotics.

First rule out the worst-case scenario

Everyone is influenced by what he or she sees most often or most recently. When dealing with a resident presentation, nurses must learn how to rule out the most lethal possible cause first.

One way is to indicate a resident condition seen frequently on the unit or department where the nurses in the particular class work, such as a resident returning to the nursing home after a right total hip replacement. Ask the attendees what is essential for the nurse to do today. Common responses will likely include to manage the pain, assess bowel and breath sounds, and verify PT is initiated.

Next ask what are the worst-case scenarios (i.e., most lethal complications) that could happen with this resident. How would you know if the resident was having those conditions? Discuss pulmonary embolism, severe anemia (requiring transfusion), aspiration pneumonia, sepsis, loss of circulation to the leg, location of the prostethesis, or a secondary condition (myocardial infarction). Often, just the technique of bringing known material into the nurses' conscious awareness helps the process become second nature.

Use test questions and illustrative stories

Another strategy is to use test questions related to a resident presentation, and find out whether nurses assess for the worst-case scenario.

Question: A 96-year-old resident admitted with pneumonia is found crawling out of the bed. What should nurses do first?

    a. Assess the resident's pain level.

    b. Obtain a pulse oximeter reading.

    c. Call for an order for a sedative.

    d. Apply a Posey jacket.

Chapter 3

Answer:

Before you give the correct answer, B, talk about residents' inability to compensate and how the brain is the most sensitive indicator for most things (low glucose, cerebral edema, etc.) Discuss whether they would feel tempted to answer differently if the person was 50 years old. Is the stereotype about all elderly people being a little confused influencing them?

Continue the lesson with a further illustration: A student nurse was told by another nurse to restrain the elderly person, which he did, but then the student nurse checked the pulse oximeter on his own. The resident was 86%.

Another true example of the danger of assuming all elderly people are confused: A resident's daughter stated her mother was more confused than usual. Though the resident's pulse oximeter was 90%, no action was taken till the resident had a small stroke the next day. Diagnostics tests then revealed a small pulmonary embolism and a new stroke caused by a second clot.

Students remember stories—use them to get your point across.

New graduate nurses and more-experienced nurses who lack critical-thinking skills tend to focus on the immediate task and orders rather than what should be done in the bigger picture. They fear acts of commission, such as giving the wrong medication. In doing so, they often commit acts of omission—not doing what they should do.

To train nurses to focus on the bigger picture, start with common situations and discuss as a group what nurses should do:

- The resident has decreased pulses in his or her leg after a knee replacement. The nurse calls the resident, who reassures the nurse that the situation is fine. What should the nurse do when obtaining the same assessment two hours later?
- The resident has neuro checks ordered every two hours. The checks have been fine for the previous eight hours. It is now 2:00 a.m. and the resident is sleeping. What should the nurse do?

Often, inexperienced nurses focus on "assessing" because they are told to assess before acting. However, emphasize the need to act when they sense through assessment that something serious is wrong. Examples of actual legal cases help illustrate this point:

- A nurse charted that the resident's pulse remained 120 all night every hour on the hour, but did nothing (until the resident coded from internal hemorrhage).

- A nurse did not wake up the resident for a neuro assessment since the ABCs were stable, and the resident had some paralysis the following morning.

- A resident's pulse oximeter remained 80% after the physician checked the resident at 1:00 a.m. The resident coded at 6:00 a.m. with respiratory acidosis.

State how important it is to at least tell somebody. Emphasize that it is all right if nurses do not know the etiology or what treatment should be given. Discuss options if one person doesn't respond (such as the charge nurse, a colleague, the nursing supervisor, another resident, the attending physician, etc.).

Role-play what nurses should say in such situations, and remember that a little humility can go a long way. As Sylvia Rayfield (2002) suggests, start with "Help me to understand . . ."

Classroom processes

Repetition is the mother of all learning
Regardless of the style, new material needs reinforcement, and this is especially important for new graduates, as the anxiety of being new adds to the need to hear things more than once. When you teach, say something again, in a slightly different way. Use personal anecdotes, legal cases, or even published literature to illustrate the principle, emotions, and consequences of the lesson. The repetition and variety of methods are penetrating.

Use unfolding case scenarios
This technique is another way to incorporate the process of clinical critical thinking in a classroom setting. It provides the information in staggered amounts, punctuated by questions. The following are examples you can use.

A resident complains of being more tired and short of breath. The resident has peripheral edema with pitting in both feet. An inexperienced nurse might focus on the swollen feet and suggest elevating the feet rather than further assessing for possible congestive heart failure.

Chapter 3

A resident fell three weeks ago and was sent for an x-ray of the right hip and spine. The resident would get in a wheelchair and go to the dining room, activities, and mass prior to the fall. Now the resident refuses to get out of bed or be turned. What would the attendees need to ask?

Remind nurses that they should conduct further assessment as to the reason for refusal. This question was based on a real-life scenario. When the nurse assessed the resident, the left leg was shorter than the right leg and externally rotated. X-ray revealed a left hip fracture requiring surgery.

Instructional approach and style

Cooperative learning

A growing trend in education is to have students teach students because "he who teaches, learns the most." One way to do this is the "think, pair, and share" exercise. Learners are given the general question and provided one minute to think about it and write down their thoughts. The task could be something like, "What are the three most important things to assess for in the first day on an abdominal postoperative resident?" or "What is something that makes it easier to delegate to an aide?"

After the minute is up, the participants then pair up and share their answers. Require each person to verbalize their thoughts to their partner, rather than just agreeing with the first person's statements. After time to share, one person is chosen as the spokesperson for the duo. Use a random selector to decide who shares, such as the person with the earliest birthday in the year, so both pay attention during the sharing.

Have the spokespeople stand and randomly select a few to repeat information from the paired sharing. Another way to change the selection is to use a version of musical chairs, passing a blown-up balloon, or have everyone stand and sit down according to certain criteria.

The advantage of a "think, pair, and share" exercise is that everyone participates. It accommodates those learners who initially need more time to think or have trouble speaking before others. They have rehearsed what they will say and can choose to enhance their response with their partners' comments. You also facilitate interaction with the material because participants must conceive it, write it, speak it, hear it, and work with it.

Multisensory learning

Most learning occurs through visual means, then hearing, with some touch. We all have our preferred style, but everyone will learn best when the logical left side and artistic right side of the brain are engaged.

Make sure your class varies the methods used to ensure multisensory learning. It's been shown that retention goes up to 50% when you hear and see something.

Effective use of discussion questions for class interaction

Throughout all discussions, pose good questions to stimulate thinking. Questions include: How does that work? What does that mean? What is the worst-case scenario here? What else do you need to know to make a decision? What makes this presentation different from the ordinary presentation? What do you want to do next? Why?

Another tip is to use silence. It can be tempting to jump in with the answer to fill the quiet (often awkward) moment that follows after a question. Train yourself to wait 10 seconds to allow time for the learners to respond. Tell the audience why you are waiting. Literally count off your fingers because 10 seconds can seem like an eternity.

It can be particularly effective to wait and not respond even when the right answer is given. This prevents learners from becoming good at reading the instructor rather than thinking about the issue. Alternatives include confirming the answer but asking the person to defend it, or to play the devil's advocate with the correct answer.

In the teaching scenarios, break the information down to what is essential, and also compare similarities or differences with a known concept. "How is this different from . . . ?"

Exude passion, as well as purpose

William Arthur Ward said, "The mediocre teacher tells. The good teacher explains. The superior teacher demonstrates. The great teacher inspires." The key behind great, effective teaching is not knowledge or methodology. It is holding a genuine passion for the material and for teaching.

Chapter 3

When teaching, pull in emotion: We often forget what we think, but almost always remember how something made us feel. The teacher's excitement and belief about the material and its importance is infectious. The learner will either catch it or (at least) respect it.

REFERENCES

Raines, C. 2002. "Managing generation X employees" in P. G. Zimmermann, *Nursing Management Secrets*. Philadelphia: Hanley & Belfus.

Rayfield, S., and L. Manning. 2002. *Nursing Made Insanely Easy!*, 3rd ed. Gulf Shore, AL: ICAN.

Salter, C. 2001. "16 ways to be a smarter teacher." *Fast Company* 53: 114–126.

Shore, D. A., and P. G. Zimmerman. 1997. "Marketing your continuing education program." *Journal of Emergency Nursing* 23 (4): 363–366.

Zimmermann, P. G. and R. D. Herr. 2006. *Triage Nursing Secrets*. St. Louis: Mosby/Elsevier.

Zimmermann, P. G. 2006. "Writing effective test questions to measure triage competency: Tips for making a good triage test." *Journal of Emergency Nursing* 32 (1): 106–109.

Zimmermann, P. G. 2006. "Education and training for triage nurses." In P. G. Zimmermann and R. D. Herr, *Triage Nursing Secrets*. St. Louis: Elsevier.

Zimmermann, P. G. 2003. "Orienting ED nurses to triage: Using scenario-based test-style questions to promote critical thinking." *Journal of Emergency Nursing* 29 (3): 256–258.

Zimmermann, P. G. 2003. "Some practical tips for more effective teaching." *Journal of Emergency Nursing* 29 (3): 283–286.

Zimmermann, P. G. 2002. "Guiding principles at triage: Advice for new triage nurses." *Journal of Emergency Nursing* 28 (1): 24–33.

Zimmermann, P. G. 2002. "The difference between teaching nursing students and registered nurses." *Journal of Emergency Nursing* 28 (6): 574–578.

SOURCES FOR EXAMPLE CASES

Legal case of the month from the Nurses Service Organization, available at *www.nso.com/case*

Triage Column/Case Review/Clinical Educator in the *Journal of Emergency Nursing*

Glendon, K., and D. Ulrich. 2001. *Unfolding Cases: Experiencing the Realities of Clinical Nursing Practice*. Upper Saddle River, NJ: Prentice Hall.

> **FIGURE 3.1** Teaching critical thinking—Critical-thinking course content and prioritization handout

Determining the need

Two components: history and physical assessment

History

Be disciplined to be consistent and thorough. Consider using a mnemonic.

POSHPATE: History of the chief complaint (Rutenberg, C. 2000. "Telephone triage." *American Journal of Nursing* 100 (3): 77–78, 80–81.)

P	Problem
O	Onset
S	Associated symptoms
H	Previous history
P	Precipitating factors
A	Alleviating/aggravating factors
T	Timing
E	Etiology

- Document key findings that allowed you to rule out the worst-case scenario or that made you think there was a problem.
- Compare to the resident's normal, especially for a chronic or elderly condition. ("You look like you are having a little trouble breathing. Is that how you are feeling?")
- Your concern should be heightened if the resident is concerned enough to complain about an "ordinary" condition (e.g., headache).

Assess before acting

Question: A resident is admitted to the nursing home after a total left knee replacement. The resident complains of pain. Nurses should first:

    a. Administer the PRN analgesic
    b. Assess for bowel sounds
    c. Obtain a description of the pain including location
    d. Chart vital signs

Answer: **C.** Do not assume the pain is related to the knee replacement. There could be a pulmonary embolism or a deep-vein thrombosis. Assess location for swelling and shortness of breath.

Chapter 3

| FIGURE 3.1 | Teaching critical thinking—Critical-thinking course content and prioritization handout (cont.) |

Prioritization with individual residents

Maslow

Self-actualization needs

Esteem needs

Safety needs

Physiologic needs

ABCD: A before B before C before D

A	Airway	If the resident is talking, the airway is intact
B	Breathing	Normal respirations are quiet and effortless
C	Circulation	Pink, warm, orientation r/t perfusion
D	Disability	Pain
		Neurological assessment
		Mental status changes

Quick Tip: 30-2-CAN DO means resident is adequately oxygenated and perfused to allow you to proceed. (Respirations are less than 30; resident is oriented to person and place, and obeys commands.)

Among ABCD, level of severity is considered.

Question: All of these residents complain of being short of breath. Which resident should nurses provide care to first?

    a. Resident with bronchitis who can speak phrases

    b. Resident with emphysema with a PO2 of 92% on 2L/min

    c. Resident three days postoperative with a cough productive of green phlegm

    d. Resident with asthma on whom the nurse cannot auscultate breath sounds

Answer: D

FIGURE 3.1	Teaching critical thinking—Critical-thinking course content and prioritization handout (cont.)

Airway

Risk for airway problems

- Decreased level of consciousness
- Sedated
- Vomiting
- Allergic reactions (unpredictable progression)

Signs of airway distress

- Hoarseness (after smoke inhalation, unrelated to a cold)
- Singed nasal hairs
- Snoring respirations (tongue falling back in an unconscious resident)
- Presence of vomitus, bleeding, secretions
- Edema of the lips/mouth tissues
- Preferred position (tripod)
- Drooling in an adult (throat epiglottis is too swollen to swallow spit,)
- Dysphagia
- Abnormal signs, such as stridor, gurgling, "death rattle" from secretions

Assess

- Look, listen, feel
- Level of consciousness r/t oxygenation

Interventions

- Reposition
- Suction

Breathing

Assess

- Respiration rate AND depth
- Symmetrical chest rise and fall

Chapter 3

> **FIGURE 3.1** Teaching critical thinking—Critical-thinking course content and prioritization handout (cont.)

- Presence and quality of bilateral breath sounds
- Pulse oximeter

Signs of respiratory problems
- Increased work of breathing (nasal flaring, retractions, expiratory grunting, accessory muscle use, head bobbing)
- Paradoxical respirations
- Jugular vein distention
- Tracheal position
- Abnormal breath sounds (silent chest is the most ominous because air is not moving)
- Color, especially circumoral (cyanosis is a late sign)
- Lack of integrity in chest wall
- Speaks in words, phrases, incomplete sentences

Related routine aspects to assess
- Is oxygen on properly, correct amount?
- Peak flow
- Resident's self-rating on the work of the breathing (Borg scale)

Interventions
- Position
- Oxygen
- Ventilation

Circulation
Assess
- Skin color, temperature
- Perfusion through blanching, capillary refill
- Pulse: rate, rhythm characteristics

FIGURE 3.1	Teaching critical thinking—Critical-thinking course content and prioritization handout (cont.)

General rule of thumb: Adults with a radial pulse have ≥ 80 systolic (brachial ≥ 70; jugular ≥ 60); low perfusion; respiratory and heart rate increase first, before blood pressure

Blood pressure: Adults must lose about 1500cc of volume before hypotension onsets

Signs of circulation difficulties
- Early signs and symptoms: loss of consciousness (LOC)
- Uncontrolled bleeding: spurting = arterial
- Distended jugular veins
- Distant heart tones
- Pitting dependent edema: pedal, sacral in a bedridden resident
- Most frequent sign of deep-vein thrombosis: unilateral extremity swelling
- Neurovascular (5 Ps)
    - Paresthesia is the early sign; nerves are more sensitive than pulse

Interventions
- IV
    - Is the site intact?
    - Is the dressing intact?
    - Is the infusion "working" at the proper rate?
- Drainage
    - Dressing dry and intact?
- Circulation devices (foot pumps, SCDs, TED hose properly applied)

Disability
Assess
- Alteration of orientation x 3 (scales)
- Alertness
- Neuro checks (Glasgow Coma Scale, PERRLA, movement/strength in all extremities)

Chapter 3

| FIGURE 3.1 | Teaching critical thinking—Critical-thinking course content and prioritization handout (cont.) |

- Pain
  - Objective score.
  - PQRST.
  - Effect on normal ADL.
  - More concern if the pain wakes the resident up, reaches maximum intensity in the first minute, resident can recall the exact moment it started suddenly, or is similar to the pain the resident had for a serious etiology (e.g., "This feels like the last time I had a heart attack.").
  - If resident states it is the "worst pain in my life" but appears comfortable or has a minor complaint (e.g., sore throat), ask about the person's previous worst pain experience. Any experience is the worst the first time you have it. If compared to significant event, such as childbirth, kidney stone, or broken bone, then accept it.

Assessment guidelines
Consider and rule out the worst-case scenario resident could have with this complaint.

What area or problem is most likely to result with this resident's condition?

Facial surgery	Airway/breathing
Broken arm	Compartment syndrome, loss of circulation
Diabetes mellitus	Hypoglycemia, DKA, HHNK
Fall	Head injury; fracture

Question: What assessment is important for a resident with a pressure ulcer?

      a. Albumin
      b. Wound stage
      c. Mobility
      d. All of the above

Answer: D

The critical-thinking classroom

FIGURE 3.1 Teaching critical thinking—Critical-thinking course content and prioritization handout (cont.)

Question: A resident returns four days postoperative from abdominal surgery. Today the resident has a temperature of 103.1°F (39.5°C), 104/60, 110/20. This morning's WBC results are 20,000. It is most important for nurses to:

    a. Administer a PRN antipyretic
    b. Monitor the vital signs every hour
    c. Assess for bowel sounds
    d. Call the physician for antibiotics

Answer: D

Go for the most common problem first. "When you hear hoof beats, think horses, not zebras."

The resident presents with a forearm deformity from falling three hours ago. He complains of severe pain.

What is the most likely explanation? Pain from a fracture.
What must be ruled out? Compartment syndrome, loss of circulation.
How will you assess this? 5 Ps; passive stretching, if relief obtained from analgesic.

Residents before paperwork.

Stop any procedure causing harm.

Question: While the nurse is administering an IV antibiotic, the resident becomes flushed and complains of feeling hot. The nurse should first:

    a. Complete an Adverse Drug Reaction form
    b. Call the doctor for an order for an antihistamine
    c. Stop the infusion
    d. Check the client's allergic history

Answer: C

Chapter 3

| FIGURE 3.1 | Teaching critical thinking—Critical-thinking course content and prioritization handout (cont.) |

Question: The charge nurse notices the new nursing assistant placing the resident's urine Foley bag on a hook at the height of the resident's chest. What is the best response for the nurse to make?

    a. Move the bag and speak to the assistant now.
    b. Speak to the assistant at the end of the shift.
    c. Discuss the need for additional inservicing with the nurse educator.
    d. Write an incident report and inform the nurse manager.

Answer: A

Medications tend to be a priority, especially for antidiabetic and antibiotic medications because of the lack of effectiveness if not given in a timely manner.

Consider the timing/type of medication
Two antibiotics are ordered for 1:00 p.m. One is every 24 hours, one is every four hours. The nurse should administer the one ordered every four hours first at 1:00 pm to allow for the best interval.

Question: A nurse had been involved with an emergency and is late in administering the team's 9:00 a.m. medications. Which of the 9:00 a.m. medications is most important for the nurse to administer first?

    a. Ampicillin 1000 mg IVPB every six hours
    b. Vancomycin 1 gram IVPB every 36 hours
    c. Lanoxin (digoxin) 0.125 mg daily
    d. Aspirin 81 mg daily

Answer: A

Question: A nurse was involved with another resident's cardiac arrest and is behind schedule with medications. It is now 8:00 a.m. Which medication is most important?

    a. Colace
    b. Ferrous sulfate
    c. Erythromycin po
    d. 70/30 insulin

Answer: D

| FIGURE 3.1 | Teaching critical thinking—Critical-thinking course content and prioritization handout (cont.) |

Prioritization principles

Acute before chronic.

Question: Which of the following residents is most important for the nurse to follow up with first?

    a. Reports unilateral blurry central vision for one year

    b. States has a veil starting to come across the vision in one eye

    c. Yellow discharge noted from right eye, relates had it for one day

    d. Complains of itching eyes during the spring

Answer: B

Sudden onset is usually more serious than gradual onset. Actual over potential.

Trends

- **Any symptom associated with other definitive changes** (e.g., not feeling well, and a fever, and feeling short of breath)
- **Any minor symptoms that tend to recur repeatedly or intensify in severity** ("nagging" cough that won't go away, smoker)
- **Steady progressive decline**

Question: Which resident with these findings is most important for the nurse to check on first?

    a. Respirations: 16, 18, 20

    b. Radial pulse: 80, 86, 92

    c. Blood pressure: 150/80, 130/78, 110/70

    d. Pulse oximeter: 99%, 97%, 96%

Answer: C

Life before limb (systemic before local).

Critical Thinking in Long-Term Care Nursing

Chapter 3

| FIGURE 3.1 | Teaching critical thinking—Critical-thinking course content and prioritization handout (cont.) |

Question: Which resident should the nurse take care of first?

    a. Resident with a leaking catheter

    b. Resident with deep-vein thrombosis complaining of shortness of breath.

    c. Resident with low-back pain complaining that it radiates down the right leg.

    d. Resident with chronic arterial insufficiency complaining of leg pain while walking.

Answer: B

Resident demographics

Presence of other risk factors increase this resident's priority

- Elderly (decreased immunity, decreased reserves to fight other stresses)
- Altered immunity (leukemia, HIV+ or AIDS, taking steroids, splenectomy)
- Multiple comorbidities (especially diabetes because less immunity)
- Reaction that has a potential to worsen (overdose, allergic response)

Avoid exposure of susceptible individuals.

Question: The skilled nursing facility will receive a new admission from the emergency department diagnosed with methicillin-resistant Staphylococcus aureus (MRSA). Which of the following residents would be the best choice for a roommate?

    a. A resident with a draining pressure ulcer

    b. A resident with bacterial pneumonia

    c. Another resident with MRSA

    d. Consider a private room

Answer: C

Remember a "known" resident can develop a new problem.

FIGURE 3.1	Teaching critical thinking—Critical-thinking course content and prioritization handout (cont.)

Avoid the "Oh my GOD!" distracter (red herring)
Remember to avoid WHO rather than "what."

Just because someone is more demanding or "ranked" higher, they should not distract from a more urgent resident need. Express your limit. "I understand you need me. I have to take care of this urgent need first and then I can work with you."

Question: Which of the following should the nurse take care of first?

   a. The bathroom sink has a leak.
   b. An irate family member is in the hall, demanding to see the supervisor.
   c. A resident is lying on the floor, having fallen and hit her head.
   d. A physician is at the nurses' station and wants to discuss an order.

Answer: C

Remember, prioritization does not mean a person's need is not met. It means first things first so the right care is given to the right person at the right time for the right reason.

Source: Polly Gerber Zimmermann, RN, MS, MBA, CEN

Chapter 3

| FIGURE 3.2 | Teaching critical-thinking skills—Sample course content, objectives, and scenarios |

Sample course objectives

1. Identify four mechanisms or thought processes that are examples of critical thinking.
2. List two validations for the need of accurate baseline assessments.
3. Describe the nursing home policy on resident reassessments.
4. Relate an atypical geriatric patient scenario that involves the cardiopulmonary system.
5. Identify two medications commonly prescribed to the geriatric patient that may mask signs/symptoms of shock.
6. Relate two responsibilities of the nurse that require critical-thinking skills.
7. Describe the use of pertinent negatives and positives in nursing documentation.

Sample course content

- Patient assessment
    - Reviewing collected data and making a decision
    - Using pertinent negatives and positives
    - Common errors
    - How vital are vital signs?

- Documentation
    - When to document
    - What not to document
    - Where to document

- When to call the physician
    - Age-specific concerns

- Red flags of assessment
    - Case scenarios

- Incorporating policy and procedure

FIGURE 3.2 Teaching critical-thinking skills—Sample course content, objectives, and scenarios (cont.)

- Professional responsibilities
  - Scope of practice
  - Risk management

Sample scenarios for student workbook or discussion

Case 1

Temp 97.4° (rectal)   Pulse 118   Respirations 26   Blood Pressure 128/72

Which vital sign is not only out of the normal range, but of most concern to you?

What are you concerned about with this resident?

What should you assess on this patient to determine if there is a potential for demise?

Case 2

Temp 102.4° (oral)   Pulse 78   Respirations 14   Blood Pressure 78/52

In the resident, what is of concern to you with these vital signs?

What other information do you need to determine if there is a potential for demise?

Source: Shelley Cohen, RN, BS, CEN

Chapter 3

> ### FIGURE 3.3 — Teaching critical-thinking skills—Classroom tips
>
> **1. Incorporate anatomy and physiology**
> - Hand out crayons or colored pencils
> - Use applicable anatomy sheets from www.enchantedlearning.com
> - Display (via slide or poster) the anatomy section you want students to fill in
> - Identify a specific area (for example, the brain) and have students color it a certain color
> - When completed, display a correct completed anatomy picture and have learners self-correct their drawings
>
> **2. Incorporate policy and procedures**
> - Identify policy/procedure appropriate to case scenarios you are using
> - Ask if students know where to retrieve/access the policy/procedure
> - Emphasize standards of practice
>
> **3. Case scenarios**
> - Use as many as you can fit into the time period
> - If multiple specialty areas are in the class, vary the scenarios
> - Relate critical-thinking strategies as you go through the cases
>
> **4. Documentation**
> - Use your standard nursing documentation forms or a printout of your electronic form
> - Give students a case scenario and have them document the resident assessment
> - Go around the room and have a few participants read their charts
> - Display a correct documentation note for the resident case
> - Discuss risk-management concerns related to documentation
>
> **5. Resources**
> - If you can access the Internet in your classroom setting, search for clinical scenarios that have photos (e.g., a rash, lab results) and pose questions to the participants
> - Use tools such as crossword puzzles to help participants improve their prioritizing skills

FIGURE 3.3 — Teaching critical-thinking skills—Classroom tips (cont.)

6. Evaluation

Obtain feedback from participants to determine if they would like a follow-up to this critical-thinking-skills course. Give them course content options and let them check off which they are interested in:

- More anatomy and physiology
- Laboratory results
- IV fluids
- Critical situation scenarios
- Interventions for an emergency

7. Self-assessment tools

Incorporate a self-assessment tool that participants can complete and use to work with preceptors or managers (Figure 3.4). Consider having participants complete the same form before and after the class to validate the need for the course and to show them how attending has improved their critical-thinking skills.

Source: Shelley Cohen, RN, BS, CEN

FIGURE 3.4 — Teaching critical-thinking skills—Sample self-assessment tool

Use the following scale to respond to each statement:

- **4** = I feel very comfortable with this
- **3** = I feel somewhat comfortable with this
- **2** = I feel somewhat uncomfortable with this
- **1** = I feel very uncomfortable with this

1. Calling the physician at 3 a.m. regarding a resident's status	4	3	2	1
2. Identifying a resident at risk for an immediate demise	4	3	2	1
3. Initiating emergency measures until help arrives	4	3	2	1
4. Relating changes in vital signs to the individual resident scenario	4	3	2	1
5. Knowing when to bring a resident-care concern to the attention of the charge nurse/team leader	4	3	2	1
6. Identifying age-specific red flags that would alert me to reassess the resident	4	3	2	1
7. Knowing what to document and what not to document	4	3	2	1
8. Identifying resident situations that may be a risk for myself or the organization	4	3	2	1
9. Verbally relaying to another professional my concerns regarding a resident's status	4	3	2	1

Source: Shelley Cohen, RN, BS, CEN

The critical-thinking classroom

FIGURE 3.5 — Teaching critical-thinking skills—Handout

Sample pocket card. Print out, fold in half, laminate (if possible), and give to attendees of the critical-thinking class.

Attributes of a critical thinker	When to call the physician
• Asks pertinent questions • Assesses statements and arguments • Is curious about things • Listens to others and is able to give feedback • Looks for evidence or proof • Examines problems closely • Can reject information that is not relevant or is incorrect • Wants to find the solution • Thinks independently • Questions deeply • Has intellectual integrity • Is confident in rationale for actions • Analyzes arguments • Evaluates evidence and facts • Explores consequences before taking action • Recognizes a contradiction • Evaluates policy	• Perfusion problem • Pain issue • Standing-order concern • Atypical presentation complaints • Risk-management potential • What's going in isn't coming out • Negative response to intervention • Social concerns/family issues affecting resident care

Reference: Ferrett, S. 1997. *Peak Performance: Success in College and Beyond.* New York: McGraw-Hill.

Source: Shelley Cohen, RN, BS, CEN

Chapter 4
Orientation: Bringing critical thinking to the clinical environment

By Polly Gerber Zimmermann, RN, MS, MBA, CEN

LEARNING OBJECTIVES

After reading this section, the participant should be able to:
- Determine ways to evaluate nurses' progress in critical thinking throughout orientation
- Develop strategies for the development of critical-thinking skills during the orientation process

Moving from the classroom to the bedside

As educators and nurse leaders start to think about developing a process to move teaching critical thinking from the classroom to the work setting, consider these questions:

- Can nurses who learn critical thinking in the classroom setting apply it in the clinical environment?

- How do you evaluate their ability to apply this knowledge?

- Does your orientation process incorporate critical thinking and how you do a baseline assessment on the new staff you hire?

- Are experienced nursing staff given the education they need so they may learn to identify key opportunities to develop critical thinking in your new staff?

If you focus on critical thinking from the beginning of orientation through to the annual review process, nurses will understand the vital role it plays in delivering safe resident care. Incorporating critical thinking into ongoing orientation processes allows you to build a nursing culture that embraces the concept of critical thinking from the date of hire.

Chapter 4

FIGURE 4.1 Critical-thinking self-assessment tool—General nursing skills

Employee name: _____ Date of hire: _____

Position hired for: _____

This self-assessment tool will help guide your preceptor and manager throughout your orientation process to ensure we provide you with the tools and resources you need for success.

How comfortable are you at doing the things listed below?

	I feel very comfortable with this	I feel somewhat comfortable with this	I feel somewhat uncomfortable with this	I feel very uncomfortable with this	Comments
Calling the doctor at 3:00 a.m. about a resident's status					
Identifying a resident at risk for immediate demise					
Initiating emergency measures until help arrives					
Identifying possible causes of vital sign changes related to the resident's condition					
Knowing when to bring a resident-care concern to the attention of the charge nurse, supervisor, or director of nursing					
Identifying age-specific alerts that indicate the resident needs reevaluation					
Knowing what to document and what not to document					
Identifying resident scenarios that may be a risk-management concern					
Verbally relaying concerns to another professional					

Source: Shelley Cohen, RN, BS, CEN

Beginning with orientation

When you mention orientation to new nursing staff members, they typically think of sitting in a classroom to learn specifics about your organization. They expect you to address medication policies, fire safety, and The Joint Commission standards, among other regulatory requirements. They also expect to take a medication test to validate that they can apply their skills in the clinical arena.

Since nurses know these items will be addressed as part of the orientation process, this is an ideal setting to introduce your expectations on critical-thinking abilities, both for new graduate nurses and for those with more experience.

Self-assessment

Once orientees have undergone classroom education regarding critical thinking, they will naturally conduct their own internal review of the information to figure out how well they function with the concepts. It is to be expected that new graduate nurses will demonstrate the most hesitancy in this area.

Regardless of the years of experience of your new hires, conducting a self-assessment is a valuable tool to measure their perception of their ability to perform at the critical-thinking level. Figure 4.1 is an example of a tool that can be used to measure nurses' critical thinking skills for general nursing responsibilities. Figure 4.2 is tailored for long-term care nursing skills. Give either or both of these forms to new hires to complete at the start of orientation. The forms should be reviewed by the new hires and their preceptors, and occasionally even their managers.

Chapter 4

FIGURE 4.2 — Critical-thinking self-assessment tool—Long-term care nursing skills

Employee name: _____ Date of hire: _____

Position hired for: _____

This self-assessment tool will help guide your preceptor and manager throughout your orientation process to ensure we provide you with the tools and resources you need for success.

How comfortable are you at doing the things listed below?

	I feel very comfortable with this	I feel somewhat comfortable with this	I feel somewhat uncomfortable with this	I feel very uncomfortable with this	Comments
Identifying red flags that a resident is no longer stable					
Defining my role when a resident has a critical lab value					
Making a decision at initial assessment that reflects the seriousness of the resident's condition					
Anticipating needs of residents presenting with acute exacerbations of chronic illnesses such as CHF, DM, or HTN					
Identifying signs and symptoms of potential abuse					
Recognizing signals that a resident or visitor has the potential for violent behavior					
Communicating long-term care regulations with the physician					
Assisting with the care of a recently deceased resident and his/her family					

Orientation: Bringing critical thinking to the clinical environment

FIGURE 4.2 — Critical-thinking self-assessment tool—Long-term care nursing skills (cont.)

	I feel very comfortable with this	I feel somewhat comfortable with this	I feel somewhat uncomfortable with this	I feel very uncomfortable with this	Comments
Preparing the family of a resident for news that will not be well received					
Caring for a resident with a fall					
Caring for a resident with a pressure ulcer					
Assessing a resident for elopement potential					
Feeding a resident via a feeding tube					
Care planning—acute, chronic					
Dealing with chronic pain					

Source: Shelley Cohen, RN, BS, CEN, and Kelly A. Goudreau, DSN, RN, CNS-BC

When developing your own self-assessment tool, or adapting the ones included, make sure to include items that reflect:

- Generic nursing skill
- Specialty-area questions
- Questions for both the novice and experienced nurse

New hires should be asked to complete the same self-assessment tools when they conclude their orientation period, or after about three months. You can then compare the responses to the initial assessment, which also could be reviewed by the preceptor and/or manager. Keep in mind that the responses may show no difference when the experience or knowledge level of nurses is at its peak performance level. Others should show marked improvements during this period, particularly new graduate nurses.

Chapter 4

Having new employees conduct a self-assessment at the beginning of orientation and again after they have been at your facility for a few months helps by:

- Clarifying and defining their critical-thinking abilities and identifying areas that require more attention during orientation
- Providing a documentation process that validates areas of strength and weakness
- Becoming a resource tool from which you and the nurse may develop goals
- Providing a record of the dates that orientees demonstrated these proficiencies

The role of preceptors

As new hires transition through the orientation process, their assigned preceptors will be key to the application of critical thinking in the clinical practice area. Regardless of experience level, new hires will look to their preceptors as role models for critical-thinking skills.

Before preceptors can teach critical thinking to orientees, they must first be practicing the skills themselves. Therefore, make sure you pick clinically competent critical thinkers who will be suitable role models for the type of nursing care you want practiced. It is also important that the organization invest time and education in training preceptors so they can meet your expectations.

Preceptors should be provided with guidelines and goals to follow as they orient new employees. This will help them to:

- Validate successful goals in the new hire
- Clearly identify areas that require remediation
- Present organized documentation to show that the new hire is able to meet the requirements of the job for which they were hired

New hires who quickly display critical-thinking skills will bring a great sense of relief to their preceptors. All new hires should display skills as they progress through their development, but those who show evidence earlier than others take quite a load off the mind of the preceptor.

Orientation: Bringing critical thinking to the clinical environment

How can preceptors teach critical thinking?

Preceptors can help orientees develop and stimulate the use of critical-thinking skills by following some of these suggestions.

How can preceptors teach critical thinking?

Minimize the emphasis on ability to perform skills and tasks: New hires are eager to complete the required "check-offs" for competencies related to performing clinical tasks. Preceptors should encourage them to focus on other aspects of their orientation as well, for example, finding the facility's policy on dealing with residents who want to leave AMA.

Maximizing emphasis on the ability to recognize when the skill or task is needed: As new hires request to be "checked off" on various skills or tasks, preceptors should ask questions to demonstrate whether new hires have the ability to critically think through why the resident needs this particular task or skill performed.

Encourage a realistic time frame and expectations: Display time-related goals for the new hire so the peer group will not have unrealistic expectations of when the new hire will be comfortable with something. Post a spreadsheet that lists the names of the orientees and goals for the next 30 days. Affix dates to the items so preceptors may check them off when successfully completed. This serves to keep all staff up to date on what orientees are competent to do, and ensures they do not delegate a task for which an orientee is not yet prepared. It also keeps a check on any unrealistic expectations staff nurses may have for new hires. Staff nurses can look at the list and know that orientees cannot admit a resident on their own because that skill will not be taught until the next time sheet.

Do not assume the new hire understands the what, why, how, or when of delivering nursing care: If the orientee is a seasoned nurse, the preceptor should not make assumptions that length of experience is directly related to knowledge and ability to use critical-thinking skills. Instead, all new hires should be required to demonstrate the same knowledge. The preceptor can use prompting questions to begin the what, why, how, and when questioning to allow the new hire to demonstrate appropriate reasoning.

Chapter 4

Figure 4.3 serves as a helpful guide for both the preceptor and the orientee to validate this process of finding out the what, why, how, and when.

FIGURE 4.3 — Preceptor tool—Relating skills to critical thinking for new graduate nurses

	Why does my resident need this?	How will I know if it is working?	What else should I consider/observe?	How long will my resident need it for?
Intravenous access with large-bore catheter or PICC line/central line				
Pressure ulcer prevention and care				
Medication protocol, such as for psychotropic medications or anticoagulants such as heparin or insulin				
Bed or chair alarms				
Foley catheter/urostomy, colostomy, ileostomy				
Tracheostomy care				
Suctioning				
Pain management				
Sequential compression devices (SCD) or other equipment				
Feeding tubes				
Pulse oximetry/oxygen				
Tracheostomy				
Feeding assistance/TPN/tube feeding				
Mobility assistance devices (walker, wheelchair, braces, cane)				

Source: Shelley Cohen, RN, BS, CEN; Kelly A. Goudreau, DSN, RN, CNS-BC; and Janie Krechting RN-C, BSN, MGS

Figure 4.3 serves as a helpful guide for both the preceptor and the orientee to validate this process of finding out the what, why, how, and when.

Teachable moments

Once new hires are in the clinical setting, there are numerous opportunities for the preceptor to teach and demonstrate the application of critical thinking with actual residents. This is also the time when new hires to reveal their ability to apply the knowledge they started learning in the orientation classroom.

Examples of "teachable moments" include:
- Preparation of assignment/organization during their shift
- Information shared during shift report
- Early identification of residents in need of specific interventions that can involve new hires
- Prompting the what/why/how/when questions for specific resident scenarios

Figure 4.4 is a tool to encourage the critical thinking of the orientee, and can be filled in to provide further examples of situations that present teachable moments. Adapt the problem list in this figure to include items directly related to your clinical practice area.

Chapter 4

FIGURE 4.4 Preceptor tool—Relating resident observations to critical thinking

Dealing with problems or situations

Problem or situation	What does the resident need?	Why does the resident need this?	How do I do this?	When should I do this?	What should I document? Where do I document?
Resident is identified with a new in-house pressure ulcer					
Resident falls					
The resident who just received a terminal diagnosis due to cancer shows no signs of sadness or grieving					
A resident has a critical lab value such as a PT INR of 25					
Resident is attempting to elope					
The resident's heart rate or rhythm has changed significantly over the last 24 hours					
Edema to periphery is increasing, breath sounds have crackles					
Resident's level of consciousness has changed over last 24 hours					
Resident has a sentinel event, e.g., fecal impaction, dehydration, or pressure ulcer in low-risk resident					
Resident's level of consciousness has changed over last 24 hours					

Source: Shelley Cohen, RN, BS, CEN; Kelly A. Goudreau, DSN, RN, CNS-BC; and Janie Krechting RN-C, BSN, MGS

Orientation: Bringing critical thinking to the clinical environment

Sometimes nursing staff other than the preceptor may be working with the orientee. During these times, it is essential that the preceptor educate all staff on the importance of their role in assisting with the transition process of the newly hired nurse.

The preceptor can promote and encourage positive behaviors among staff that will help to promote and motivate the critical-thinking process. Figure 4.5 is a tool preceptors can share with other staff to encourage their understanding and support for developing new employees' critical thinking. It has essential reminders that include:

- Faster is not always clinically better
- Checking things off for a new hire indicates you observed them perform it
- You should proactively involve new hires in challenging resident scenarios—but be there to support them
- You should ask prompting questions that validate whether new hires can apply knowledge
- Knowing where your department resources are is as important as learning tasks and skills

FIGURE 4.5 Preceptor tool—Promote and support critical thinking

To encourage newly hired nurses in their orientation process, we all need to provide a supportive and nurturing clinical environment. We want team members who can answer the what/why/how/when of nursing process.

Here's how you can help to create this environment.

1. Faster is not necessarily better, as long as it's done correctly

Does it really matter—in many situations—if it takes new hires a few minutes longer to get in the IV? Yes, you could have done it faster—but how fast did you do it when you were a new nurse?

2. Make no assumptions about skills

If you are asked to check off a new hire on a skill, be sure you actually observe the performance of this skill and then ask:

Critical Thinking in Long-Term Care Nursing

| FIGURE 4.5 | Preceptor tool—Promote and support critical thinking (cont.) |

- Why does/did this resident need a _____?
- How did you know the correct way to perform this?
- Where did you find the information?
- How will you tell if the procedure is helpful for the resident?
- What and where will you document what you have done?

3. **When you identify a challenging resident scenario or a procedure not commonly performed, invite the new hire to participate**

   This will help increase the experience of the new hire, as well as help the team identify the new hire's willingness to learn.

4. **At shift-change report, ask prompting questions in a nondefensive manner**
   - What do you think is going on with this resident?
   - Are you comfortable with what the provider told you after you spoke with him or her?

5. **Observe new hires' ability to prioritize and organize their assignments**
   - Is there a particular reason you have not done the preop teaching yet on Mrs. Jones?
   - You look concerned. Is everything okay? Let's go over your assignment and talk about priorities for the shift. I'd like to hear what you think are the most important issues in these residents and why.

6. **When questions arise, do new hires know where to look for the answers or are they simply expecting coworkers to tell them?**
   - I am not sure about these medicines being compatible. How could you find out?
   - When you are not sure whether a permit is needed for a procedure, where could you find that information?

Source: Shelley Cohen, RN, BS, CEN

Orientation: Bringing critical thinking to the clinical environment

Evaluating skills

As new nurses work their way through the orientation process, evaluating their ability to apply critical thinking in their clinical setting needs to be accomplished. Sometimes knowing what to do is as important as knowing what not to do. The preceptor needs evidence of new hires' abilities to assess the needs of each resident.

The following should be assessed:

- Evaluate a resident's health status: Are new hires resident assessment skills targeted to the resident's presentation?

- Identify potential scenarios based on the resident's health status: Are new hires aware of potential problems or complications this resident may be at risk for?

- Evaluate a resident's response to interventions: Are new hires performing an appropriate reassessment? Can they identify if the resident is the same, worse, or better?

- Evaluate the need for higher skill level. If resident is not responding to intervention, do new hires know what to do next?

- Take action when indicated: Can new hires initiate actions needed by residents, such as standing orders? Are they able to prioritize these actions?

Handling judgment or action errors during orientation

"In any moment of decision the best thing to do is the right thing, the next best thing is the wrong thing, and the worst thing you can do is nothing."

—Theodore Roosevelt

It is more encouraging to see orientees taking action in the clinical setting than to see them elect to do nothing about a resident situation. The fact that they are willing to do something shows they are making progress. And the reality is that an error of judgment may be made by an experienced nurse as well as a new graduate.

It's important to understand that placing an experienced nurse in a new and unfamiliar clinical specialty area creates an opportunity for judgment or action errors, just as new graduates may

Chapter 4

make errors due to their unfamiliarity with nursing. Experienced nurses who have moved to a new clinical specialty will be exposed to unfamiliar medications, procedures, and age-specific considerations.

For example, an experienced pediatric nurse who transitions to the nursing home is going into a world of very different patients. The nurse's medication dosing was very different for children than it will be for older patients. In addition, he or she will experience different situations and interactions with residents. For the most part, he or she developed close relationships with the families of the pediatric patients, but in a nursing home, the nurse will have to deal with residents who may have no families or caregivers. The nurse will have to deal with multiple, complex diagnoses in long-term care residents.

Accept that errors will occur and lay the groundwork for making sure errors are handled in the correct manner. Preceptors and the entire peer group play a large role in the recovery process when errors occur, and should help ensure that incidents become an opportunity to develop critical-thinking skills that will reduce such incidents in the future.

In addition, the response of the preceptor and peers to these scenarios will determine whether new hires feel supported during what is a challenging time for them. Nurses are often quick to "quarterback" incidents with comments about how "We would never have done that" or "I would never have done that first." Remember that orientation is a time of learning, setting goals, and identifying areas of strength and weakness. Newly hired nurses should not be left with a feeling of "being chewed up and spit out" by their peer group.

All incidents can be used as learning experiences. When errors occur, they may reveal some positive attributes about the new hire:

- The nurse was willing to be held accountable and identified the error to you
- The nurse was grateful and appreciative that you pointed out the error
- The nurse requested resources for self-learning to better understand the red flags that he or she missed with the resident
- The nurse asked questions to better understand how the resident got to this point
- The nurse sought guidance in completing a reporting form if one was needed

Preceptors or mentors of new employees must identify the decisions that were or were not made by the nurse that reflect a lack of critical thinking. Once these are recognized, then the preceptor can become the teacher to guide the nurse as he or she learns so that a similar situation is not replayed in the future.

Remediation

Working with new hires on remediation after an event is a delicate job. How you handle the situation will greatly affect how much they learn, how they feel about and whether they can accept what happened, and whether they develop their critical-thinking skills so as to understand the situation.

These teaching qualities will help you have a successful interaction:

Patience: What is obvious critical thinking to you may not be for others. You may need to provide repetition in the learning process and allow time for the nurse to digest the information before requiring him or her to demonstrate understanding.

Support: Being supportive after an error in judgment does not mean you minimize the importance of what occurred. It simply reflects that you support the nurse. Some words to use to send a supportive and reassuring message include:

- I understand you are upset about what happened with Mr. Smith
- I realize this material is all new to you—let's go over it again
- Take a step back and look at all the things you have accomplished
- Good for you for recognizing and notifying me of the error—it takes courage and strong ethics to do so

Clarification: Define in writing for the new hire what you expect of him or her in light of what has occurred. If you discussed timelines, include those in the written expectations. For the new hire who simply does not have the capacity to apply critical thinking, it is essential that your documentation reflect what happened, what steps were taken, and what improvements were expected to occur so as to validate any future employment decisions. Examples of written expectations include:

Chapter 4

- All medication doses requiring calculations will be reviewed with the preceptor prior to administration to the resident.

- There will be no further incidents of residents signing out AMA without nursing documentation that "tells the story" of these events. The orientee will develop a list of other risk-management scenarios related to the department and present these at our next scheduled orientation meeting.

Realism: Keep in mind the reality of the situation. It is not about what you learned in nursing school or when you went through orientation years ago. It is about the present situation and the circumstances and experiences of the new nurse.

- Remember that not all new grads are clinically prepared at the same level
- Review critical-thinking goals and timelines to ensure they are appropriate
- Recognize those nurses who may never be able to meet these goals successfully, and deal with the situation appropriately

Orientation sets critical-thinking expectations

The orientation process and critical thinking should go hand in hand. Orientation allows new hires to see how the critical-thinking skills they learned in the classroom can be integrated into practice. It is the foundation upon which they can build on their development from novice to expert.

Orientation: Bringing critical thinking to the clinical environment

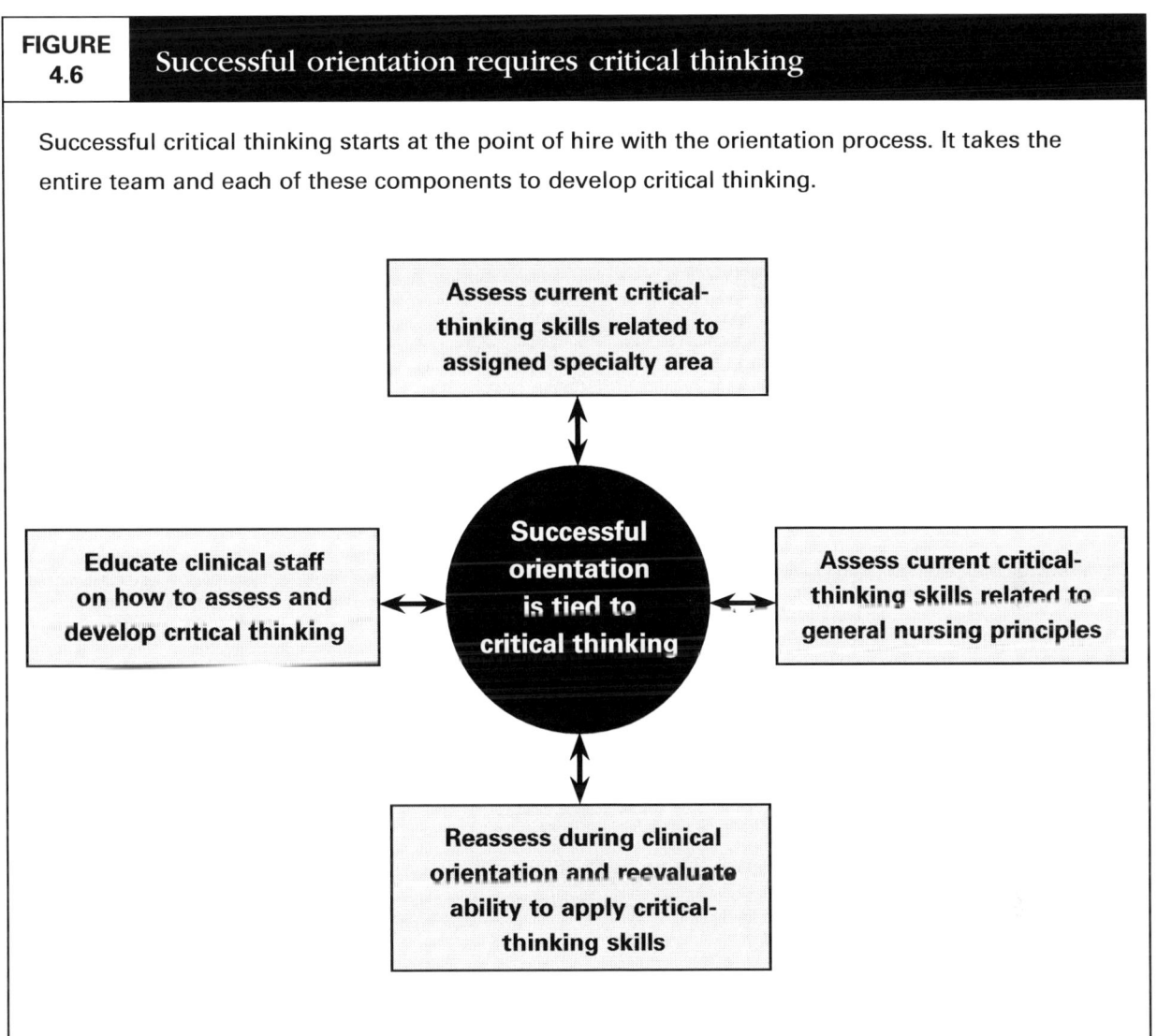

FIGURE 4.6 — Successful orientation requires critical thinking

Successful critical thinking starts at the point of hire with the orientation process. It takes the entire team and each of these components to develop critical thinking.

Source: Shelley Cohen, RN, BS, CEN

Chapter 5

Nursing practice that promotes and motivates critical thinking

By Polly Gerber Zimmermann, RN, MS, MBA, CEN

LEARNING OBJECTIVES

After reading this section, the participant should be able to:

- Discuss the role played by managers and educators in promoting environments that support critical thinking

Maintaining momentum

Once nurses have finished with orientation, the journey to critical thinking becomes more subtle.

After spending time and money to teach nursing staff about critical-thinking skills, you probably have high hopes for seeing these skills translated into improvements in resident care. Yet if you do not create an environment that supports and motivates ongoing development of critical thinking, it is unrealistic to expect most staff to continue to practice it.

Immediately after completing a course on critical thinking, most experienced nurses will independently implement critical thinking in their daily practice. But without a setting that supports the ongoing development and use of these skills, nurses will easily fall back into practice patterns that do not involve a higher level of reasoning. New graduate nurses have no previous experiences or practices to fall back on, but the reality of practice may reduce their ability to think critically. How they are mentored and the role models of experienced nurses around them will determine what they will offer for resident care.

Nurses respond well to challenging work environments and practice settings that embrace critical thinking. Nurses who practice critical thinking operate at a higher level, meaning they are more likely to be stimulated and fulfilled professionally. This may be demonstrated by:

Chapter 5

- Interest in committee involvement
- Support for quality improvement efforts
- Proactively seeking to attend ongoing education
- Initiating more collaborative efforts with other members of the team
- Early identification of acute changes in residents

In addition to the preceptor/mentor, the following people and practices play important roles in encouraging the ongoing development and implementation of critical thinking and practice standards. Identify the areas in which you can implement the most immediate change.

- Nurse manager
- Nurse educator
- Defining critical-thinking expectations in a written format through:
    - Job descriptions
    - Clinical guidelines
    - Policy and procedure

Nurse managers and staff educators

Newly hired and seasoned staff will look to nurse managers, as the leader of the department(s), to validate how much importance they should place on this "critical-thinking stuff." They will look to staff educators to provide leadership and ongoing education.

Nurse managers and staff educators should set expectations for critical thinking by expecting staff to have the ability to:

- Organize
- Prioritize
- Delegate
- Practice safely
- Apply reasoning when making decisions

Nursing practice that promotes and motivates critical thinking

These are the skills of nurses who have the ability to make appropriate decisions, and they will have been discussed through classroom sessions and during orientation. But if managers and educators do not maintain the momentum through a culture that requires ongoing development of critical thinking, your orientation efforts will fall short. You need to ensure a resident-care environment that nurtures critical thinkers, that stimulates them and motivates them to engage in a discussion in their minds. This discussion is all about one question: Is this in the best interest of the resident?

Take out one of your time sheets, and as you look down the list of names, ask yourself how you really feel about each nurse's ability to demonstrate these attributes. Use Figure 5.1 to assist you as you validate educational and remediation needs of individual staff. This tool also may be used by preceptors and senior staff—such as charge nurses—who are involved in assessing staff performance.

FIGURE 5.1 Critical-thinking skills assessment—Nurse manager/staff educator tool

Staff member name	1	2	3	4	5	6	7	8	9	10	11	12	13	14	15

1. Asks pertinent questions
2. Assesses statements/arguments
3. Displays curiosity
4. Listens to others and gives feedback
5. Looks for evidence or proof
6. Examines problems closely
7. Rejects incorrect information
8. Wants to find answers
9. Independently thinks things through
10. Displays confidence about actions
11. Can analyze an argument
12. Looks at the evidence and facts
13. Considers consequences before acting
14. Recognizes contradictions
15. Evaluates policy and considers appropriateness for patient

Source: Shelley Cohen, RN, BS, CEN

Chapter 5

Making critical thinking part of the culture

For critical thinking to be a part of your nursing culture, it has to be more than something that is simply "checked off" once a year. The concepts of reasoning should be ingrained in the following:

- Job descriptions
- Clinical guidelines
- Policy and procedure
- Performance reviews
- Processes that incorporate goal setting

Job descriptions

Job descriptions that do not reflect the reality of what staff members actually do or are expected to do provide no foundation for staff accountability, but it is impossible to include every item, task, or responsibility that nurses will be expected to perform. Therefore, using terminology related to critical thinking sends a clear message that "other duties" may be required.

To improve the content of your job descriptions, consider:

- Involving staff in the process of updating and reviewing job descriptions on a regular basis. Ask prompting questions to assist staff in this process:
    - What are you doing on a regular basis that is not on the job description?
    - What is on the job description that you no longer do?
    - What do you feel should be added that will help hold all nurses more accountable?
- Identify resident scenarios that demonstrated a lack of critical thinking:
    - Was there anything absent from the job description that made it difficult to hold staff accountable for their action or lack of action?
    - Were there practice standards related to the scenario that were not followed? If so, do the current job descriptions define the expectation that staff members are responsible for maintaining a current knowledge base for the specialty in which they provide nursing care?

Nursing practice that promotes and motivates critical thinking

> **Job description examples**
>
> - Nurses will use critical-thinking skills to determine action needed for risk management concerns such as medical restraint of residents; elopement; violent or combative resident, visitor, or family behavior; and suspected abuse or neglect.
>
> - The reassessment process for post-fall residents is dictated by policy, but nurses are expected to critically think through the specific needs of each resident and understand which residents may require more frequent monitoring than policy dictates.
>
> - Nurses will use critical-thinking skills to manage their workload and offer support to other team members as indicated by resident acuity and staff skill mix on the unit.

Clinical guidelines

We all know staff members who attend training events and seminars, yet do not have the ability to apply what they learned in the clinical setting. An example of this may be the nurse who successfully passes the written exam and the testing stations, yet he or she is disorganized and lacks knowledge in an actual resuscitative event. The same principle applies to critical-thinking concepts. The nurse may have been taught critical-thinking principles, yet when performing resident care he or she does not appear to "have it together." This may present itself as disorganization or even in an actual medical error from a lack of judgment.

Clinical guidelines—also referred to as care paths and clinical pathways—provide evidence-based interventions and direction to set standards of practice for specific resident clinical presentations. These models require the nurse to use reasoning and prioritization to determine when to take each step in the guideline. (If nurses are unable to follow clinical guidelines, they need remediation and further help.)

The implementation of clinical guidelines demonstrates the use of standards of practice, as well as implying that nurses possess the critical thinking needed to apply the guidelines.

Chapter 5

Policy and procedure

When relating policy and procedure to critical thinking, you should expect nurses to grasp the following:

- Know where policies and procedures are kept
- Read the policies and procedures
- Understand what each policy is asking/requiring
- Identify the resident/situation for which to engage each policy or procedure

---

Policy and procedure examples

Reassessment of the long-term care resident

The long-term care nurse will use critical-thinking skills when reassessing a resident across the span of an eight- or 12-hour shift. Specifically, the long-term care nurse must think in a comprehensive manner and not just on the focused area of concern. A resident's condition can change gradually over time. Small indicators are important when looked at in the context of the whole person. For this reason it is important that the nurse does a comprehensive assessment at the beginning of the shift and uses that as a baseline for any changes that may occur during the shift.

Communication of concerns to the team

It is important that long-term care nurses recognize that although they usually function on their own process and time management, they also have support systems in place. The charge nurse, supervisor, nurse manager, assistant director of nursing, or director of nursing (depending on your particular system) are there to provide support when a resident's condition appears to be changing. Communicate your questions or areas that "do not look right" to the support systems around you in a clear, concise, and to-the-point manner. You will get the assistance you need to provide the best possible care to the resident.

Performance reviews

The annual review is an opportunity for the manager to reinforce expectations regarding critical thinking with each member of the nursing staff. Again, Figure 5.1 can be used or adapted to outline areas of strength and weakness for each nurse. You also may want to have the nursing staff members perform a self-assessment of their ability to think critically prior to the annual review. Figure 5.2 is an example of a self-assessment tool.

Nursing practice that promotes and motivates critical thinking

FIGURE 5.2 — Annual performance review—Self-assessment of critical thinking

Employee name: _____ Date of hire: _____

Please rate your ability to apply critical thinking in the following areas:

- **5** = I always do this
- **4** = I do this most of the time
- **3** = I sometimes do this
- **2** = I rarely do this and realize I need to be more aware in this area
- **1** = I never do this and realize I need some help to improve on this

1. I ask pertinent questions.	5	4	3	2	1
2. I assess statements/arguments before making decisions.	5	4	3	2	1
3. I am always curious about things and want to learn.	5	4	3	2	1
4. I listen to others and give feedback.	5	4	3	2	1
5. I look for evidence or proof before doing what someone else says I should do.	5	4	3	2	1
6. I examine problems closely.	5	4	3	2	1
7. I know when information is incorrect and I reject it.	5	4	3	2	1
8. I want to find answers.	5	4	3	2	1
9. I independently think things through.	5	4	3	2	1
10. I am confident in my actions.	5	4	3	2	1
11. I can analyze an argument.	5	4	3	2	1
12. I look at the evidence and facts.	5	4	3	2	1
13. I consider consequences before acting.	5	4	3	2	1
14. I recognize contradictions.	5	4	3	2	1
15. I evaluate policy and consider its appropriateness for the resident.	5	4	3	2	1

Source: Shelley Cohen, RN, BS, CEN

Chapter 5

This self-assessment tool can be compared to the worksheet you prepared for the employee's performance review and the employee's goals for the coming year (Figure 5.3 can be used to plan short- and long-term goals), and can be specific to discuss judgment and reasoning when appropriate. Other benefits of staff members performing a self-assessment of their abilities are:

- It details specific expectations from both you and the resident
- In the process of completing the tool, questions should and will arise regarding critical-thinking concepts, prompting further discussion
- It requires nurses to consider specific resident scenarios when they have actually displayed these abilities

As you and the nurse identify areas that need improvement, first prompt the nurse to offer suggestions and resources before you do. Remember, part of your role is to coach staff members —if you provide all the answers all the time, you are stifling their critical thinking.

Goal setting

When staff members demonstrate unacceptable behavior or unsafe practices, take the opportunity to discuss the importance of critical thinking. From point of hire to annual review to daily resident care, judgment will always play a central role. When setting new goals in response to unacceptable behavior or unsafe events, relate the goals to the nurse developing better judgment and displaying higher levels of critical thinking.

Figure 5.3 is an example of a goals worksheet and Figure 5.4 contains examples of what to consider saying and how to document the conversation and conclusions reached.

Nursing practice that promotes and motivates critical thinking

| FIGURE 5.3 | Goals worksheet |

Employee name: _____ Today's date: _____
Job title: _____

Short-term goals

In the next year, I would like to do the following:

Add _____ to my job description

Take _____ continuing education classes

Work on projects related to improving _____

Long-term goals

In the next 2–5 years I would like to do the following:

Have completed _____

Make these changes in my job _____

Have accomplished _____

Obtain certification in _____

Source: Shelley Cohen, RN, BS, CEN

Chapter 5

FIGURE 5.4	Setting goals for improvement

Should Nancy present to the department late on another shift between today's date and _____ she will know that:

- An off-going shift member will be delayed
- An oncoming shift nurse will have to take an additional assignment
- Resident care will be directly affected

Nancy has the ability to critically think through the ramifications for when staff members do not present on time for their shift and she has outlined these in our meeting today.

Timothy is aware of the resources available to nurses in the department when they are in need of detailed medication information. He agrees that if he had looked up the information on _____ and applied nursing judgment, the resident would not have been given the dose.

Timothy will demonstrate appropriate nursing judgment when administering medication by:

- Using available resources in the department such as reference books or by calling the pharmacy.
- Successfully completing a written medication assessment tool, achieving a grade of 90% or better. This will be done within the next 15 days.
- Having the charge nurse check all calculations for pediatric medications for the next 30 days.
- Achieving a medication pass monitor score of 95% or above.

Source: Shelley Cohen, RN, BS, CEN

Chapter 6

Novice to expert: Setting realistic expectations for critical thinking

By Polly Gerber Zimmermann, RN, MS, MBA, CEN

LEARNING OBJECTIVES

After reading this section, the participant should be able to:

- Analyze the challenges that both new and experienced nurses face in the incorporation of critical-thinking skills in the practice setting

- Explain interventions to help both new and experienced nurses meet their managers' and preceptors' expectations for critical thinking

Setting realistic expectations

As you approach and consider methods not only to teach but also to motivate critical thinking, it is essential that your expectations meet the abilities of the nurse. The last thing you want is an environment that creates fear of critical-thinking expectations. We want staff to embrace the concept, confident in their abilities to develop their thinking and reasoning skills.

Align your expectations more with what it is realistic to expect from nurses, rather than what you hope they can do. As you set your expectations, consider each nurse's potential, opportunities to perform, opportunities to reach goals, and the outcomes you hope each nurse will achieve.

Make sure your expectations are:

- Realistic

- Supported with appropriate tools and resources

- Appropriate for the specialty area in which the nurse works

- Flexible to meet a variety of learning needs

- Clarified in writing

- Related to the performance review

Chapter 6

Novice to competent: New graduate nurses

It may seem obvious that the expectations for critical thinking displayed by new graduate nurses would not be the same as those for experienced nurses. Yet many new graduate nurses are facing peer groups who have already decided what they should/should not know. Preceptors, nurse educators, and nurse managers are the ones who must set the expectations for new graduates, not the experienced nurses on the unit. Preceptors, nurse educators, and nurse managers should be the ones who communicate the expectations for new graduates to the rest of the staff.

When new graduate nurses join the skilled nursing unit, use the opportunity for the team to consider the experience of new nurses and what new graduates have to cope with. Include the following points in the discussion to enlighten staff and help them have a better understanding of why the expectations on new graduates are different today than they were in previous decades:

- Many students today have fewer clinical opportunities than most current nurses had in school.

- Students today have to contend with a chronic shortage of nursing faculty across the country.

- Many nursing schools "teach to the boards," and great focus is placed on successful completion of the NCLEX.

- Students' limited clinical time may not have exposed them to challenging residents similar to those seen in your environment.

- In years past, nurses gained several years of experience before becoming specialty nurses. Now many enter a specialty straight out of school.

Let it be known that you will not tolerate staff members who are unwilling to accept today's realities for new graduates. Do not allow statements such as, "Back in my day we were expected to . . . " The manager, preceptor, and educator need to promptly address individuals who make such comments so the message is clear: This is unacceptable behavior. Work together to script appropriate responses that hold those individuals accountable, such as, "We are not practicing 1962 nursing care here. Are you?" Be strong, as many articles have been written about experienced nursing "eating their young."

Novice to expert: Setting realistic expectations for critical thinking

As new graduates move further along and out of their orientation period, assist in the transition from novice staff nurse to competent staff nurse by considering the following:

- Use tools that allow new graduates to self-assess their level of critical thinking
- Reevaluate decision-making skills throughout the orientation process
- Promptly clarify all questions regarding expectations
- Promote a culture and environment that encourage critical thinking
- Remember that critical thinking is a process that develops and grows throughout the career
- Bear in mind that new graduates who do not employ critical thinking in their personal lives will face the greatest challenges in incorporating it into their nursing care

Greatest challenges for new graduate nurses

Among the many challenges new graduates will face—and obstacles to the development of their critical thinking—are the residents in their care, and those residents' families, who have bad outcomes and the providers who are unwilling to collaborate with them. The first makes them ask the question, "What should I have done?" The second makes them unwilling to use their critical-thinking skills, because they feel they are not needed.

The first year after graduation is a time for education, and care must be taken that new graduates are not frightened to make a decision or feel constantly indecisive in the care they provide.

Coaching new graduates through bad resident outcomes

- Allow them to grieve through their error or omission. Whether residents are in their care for one hour or one week, in their minds, they are still "my resident."
- As nurses we tend to beat ourselves up when we make a medication or other error. After we are done whipping ourselves, we move on. New graduate nurses need time to go through a process where they review what happened and how they would approach it differently next time. Our job is to coach them away from the blame and move them toward learning experiences.
- Provide them with more than one opportunity to sit with a supportive mentor or preceptor to review the scenario that led to the resident outcome.

Chapter 6

- Make sure you are the person who debriefs the new nurses. Don't expose them to the nurse who says, "I told you this would happen if you let new grads in here."

- Even if the bad outcome was not related to something they did or did not do, they still may feel like it was their fault. Coach them that a guilt trip will not change the outcome of the scenario.

- If they are not willing to take responsibility or accountability for something they did or did not do for the resident, recognize this as a resident safety warning. These nurses will require further assessment of their critical-thinking capabilities and ongoing involvement with the nurse manager.

Growing collaborative relationships with physicians, nurse practitioners, and specialists
Working with physicians can be intimidating for new graduates if steps are not taken to develop relationships. Simple steps can help promote the new relationship and build a basis of good feeling so that both sides may build trust.

- Have someone introduce new graduates to physicians as they arrive on the unit.

- If physicians have had previous negative experiences with new graduate nurses, make time to discuss the critical-thinking training you are providing these new graduates.

- Circulate a memo to residents' physicians introducing the new graduates and briefly outlining expectations, the critical-thinking training, and the names of the preceptors.

- Ask physicians to think back to their own internships and remind them that critical thinking will develop with their support.

- Provide an opportunity for new graduates to observe a variety of long-term care nursing roles, e.g., charge nurse, supervisor, Minimum Data Set nurse, infection control nurse, and director of nursing.

- In your critical-thinking training, include scenarios that allow novice nurses to explore options for how to respond to challenging times and conversations with providers. This is part of teaching them how to respond professionally to any challenge in the healthcare environment.

Novice to expert: Setting realistic expectations for critical thinking

Growing collaborative relationships with the interdisciplinary team

New graduates also face expectations from other team members, which may include ancillary services such as radiology, respiratory therapy, laboratory, and pharmacy. Build a pattern of success for new graduates by communicating with other services:

- Dates of new graduates' arrivals and the departments/areas to which they are assigned
- Include time for new nurses to observe and understand processes related to supportive services such as x-ray, lab, and pharmacy
- Discuss the time frame of the orientation process and give a list of realistic expectations related to procuring and coordinating supportive services
- Incorporate interdisciplinary team members' skills and experiences as part of the new graduate's education by including them as faculty for classroom time

When new graduates fail to reach competent levels of critical thinking

For managers and preceptors, one of the greatest challenges is when you are confronted with newly graduated nurses who just don't seem to "get it." There will be times, despite your best efforts and resources, when the concept of critical thinking will not be grasped in a realistic time frame. This situation must be addressed promptly to be fair to the newly hired nurse, the preceptor, the staff, and, of course, the residents.

While it's important to understand the emotional elements involved for new graduate nurses, this does not change the fact that the level of nursing practice being displayed is unsafe and unacceptable. It is misleading to allow the new graduate to carry on believing that "things will just work out."

Key steps to take when new graduates are not progressing with critical-thinking development include:

- Identifying early on those new graduates who are not meeting expectations
- Defining which expectations they are not meeting and providing examples
- Offering and providing remediation with new expectations and a written timeline for meeting the expectations
- If remediation does not change nursing practice, the manager should meet with human resources to determine the next appropriate step

Chapter 6

For new graduates who continue to fail to progress, consider options such as these:

- Providing opportunity for:
    - Fewer multitasking skills
    - Fewer unplanned scenarios
    - Lower resident-assignment loads
- Extending the probationary period
- Collaborating with faculty from his or her school of nursing for mediation direction

In all of this, do not disregard your obligations to residents and the State Board of Nursing as they relate to resident safety.

Competent to expert: Experienced nurses

Many of the principles that relate to new graduate nurses also apply to those with more experience. One of the challenges with experienced nurses is that many in the peer group have higher expectations and often believe these expectations are being met, even if they have no evidence to show this. For example, they see the experienced nurse demonstrate a particular skill or task well, and then assume all the nurse's skills are at that level. This type of assumption can be dangerous, and can mean experienced nurses receive less support and training for them to develop their critical-thinking skills.

Once again, it is important to define realistic expectations for all newly hired nursing staff and establish timelines for when they should accomplish these expectations.

When experienced nurses join your unit, remind the team of the following concepts:

- Just because someone successfully completes an ACLS course does not mean he or she can function in a cardiopulmonary-arrest situation
- If team members do not share concerns related to new nurse performance with the preceptor, educator, or manager, then issues cannot be addressed
- Doing a procedure faster does not imply you understand why you are doing it
- People can "talk" a great story; the test is whether they can perform at that level
- If staff nurses don't get involved in the process of orienting newly hired nurses, we cannot truly assess their abilities to think critically and act critically

Novice to expert: Setting realistic expectations for critical thinking

In addition to experienced nurses who have just joined the unit, you should also assess and support the critical-thinking development of nurses who have long been there.

Use assessment tools such as Figures 4.1, 4.2, and 5.2 to validate the ability of experienced nurses to apply critical thinking in their practice settings. For those who are unable to demonstrate their ability, initiate a remediation process in conjunction with the nurse manager.

Handling experienced nurses who need remediation

When you are confronted with seasoned nurses who are unable to meet your expectations, consider the following:

- If a new hire, do they need a different preceptor?
- If a new hire, are they still in their probationary period?
- Is there one area in which they are unable to attain a skill, or is it an overall care issue?
- If they have been staff members for a while, how has this been handled in the past?

Your facility needs to use consistency when addressing this sensitive issue. If nurses are long past the orientation period and are not meeting critical-thinking expectations, find out how this has been handled with other nurses in the past. You may want to set a new precedent for how it will be handled in the future.

Because the ability to think critically is one that is ongoing and constantly being developed, it requires ongoing reevaluation. For example, just because the nurse you hired four years ago demonstrated good strategies in nursing care when he or she was hired does not mean he or she still practices within those same principles. Consider these elements that occur in your resident care areas:

- New procedures
- New evidence and research that demonstrate a different approach to particular diagnoses
- The multitude of new medications added to the formulary each year
- New standards of practice from regulatory agencies and authorities

Chapter 6

With this list in mind, and considering that healthcare is in constant flux, it makes sense to design a process to continually reassess nurses' ability to think critically. You can directly involve staff in this process by:

- Incorporating critical-thinking language and expectations in written documents such as:
    - Policies and procedures
    - Employee handbook
    - Clinical pathways/guidelines
    - Job descriptions
    - Performance reviews
- Having staff review these written expectations annually and offer suggestions for change
- Having staff complete self-assessment sheets (see Figures 4.1, 4.2, and 5.2)
- Requiring staff to present examples at their performance reviews of how they have displayed critical thinking in their resident care

Measuring critical thinking in daily practice

How do you know whether nurses are thinking critically in their practice? Regardless of their level of experience, once they have completed orientation and have been "checked off" you are implying they no longer need daily precepting. You are making a statement that they have demonstrated the ability to meet their job description. If you do not feel they can perform their job description/requirements independently, then the orientation process needs to be extended.

Demonstrating they can think critically is more than being checked off on being able to perform a task or procedure. Use and adapt the sample tools throughout the book—such as Figure 4.4, which assesses nurses' ability to think through what residents are telling them—to evaluate their level of performance. Using standard criteria for the evaluation will help you validate whether critical thinking is part of their nursing practice, for both experienced and inexperienced nurses.

> **Examples of demonstrating critical thinking**
>
> Long-term care nurses demonstrate critical thinking by:
>
> - Identifying early symptoms of shock
>
> - Performing a full head-to-toe physical assessment to note any changes in status from the previous assessment noted in the chart
>
> - Noting any residents who may be at risk for domestic violence or elder abuse
>
> - Evaluating the intake and output of an admitted resident
>
> - Documenting and discussing with support personnel (CNAs) any physical findings noted on assessment
>
> - Discussing with support personnel any issues they need to watch for when caring for the resident's physical needs
>
> - Identifying whether a social-work consult will be needed to discharge the resident to home or assist with adjustment to long-term placement

Chapter 7
Applying critical thinking to nursing documentation

By Polly Gerber Zimmermann, RN, MS, MBA, CEN

LEARNING OBJECTIVES

After reading this section, the participant should be able to:
- Apply critical thinking to nursing documentation

Turning critical thinking into critical writing

Critical writing is as important as critical thinking. Good documentation is a vital part of resident care, and nurses need to be able to validate in the written medical record what they did or what they chose not to do. We think of the medical record as a storybook that tells what happened to the resident from the point of entry into the healthcare system to the point of exit from the system. With all of today's risk management and legal concerns that challenge the healthcare delivery systems as well as the caregivers, it is vital to demonstrate steps and actions taken to support the resident.

Identifying a resident problem, potential consequences, and necessary actions are vital elements of critical thinking for nurses. However, without appropriate and timely documentation, there is no written record of what has occurred.

Transforming critical thinking into the written format provides:
- A legal record to support a nurse's:
    - Identification of a problem
    - Actions taken in response to the problem
    - Resident outcomes related to any intervention

Chapter 7

      - Collaboration with other members of the healthcare team

      - Compliance with nursing standards of practice

- A timetable of the events to reference as a tool in determining ongoing care and needs of the resident

- Validation of the nursing process that incorporated critical thinking

Figure 7.1 lists common charting errors you can avoid as not inductive to critical thinking.

FIGURE 7.1 — Eight common charting errors

Accurate and complete nursing documentation is essential for demonstrating compliance with standards, delivery of state-of-the-art nursing care, and the ability to communicate effectively with everyone involved in resident care. Therefore, it is important to recognize common charting mistakes and ways to educate your staff about them.

Charting mistakes can lead to allegations of negligence. The following list describes the eight most common charting mistakes, along with how and why you should avoid them.

1. Failure to document pertinent health or drug information
Nurses conducting admission assessments are responsible for acquiring all pertinent health data that will influence the plan of care. As silly as this mistake may seem, nursing admission assessments and transfer notes are often left incomplete.

Good history-taking skills are especially important during the initial admission assessment, as the assessment is important to the safety and well-being of the resident. Any health information that is not gathered when taking the history or not documented in the appropriate location on the clinical record can lead to adverse consequences.

To avoid this kind of mistake, ensure that your staff members know how to take thorough histories and focus particularly on residents who cannot communicate effectively, are poor historians, or have dementia. Remind staff members to document conversations with significant others, the transferring agency, or any other source of information. Provide them with continuing education regarding communication skills needed to ascertain a complete and thorough patient history.

Applying critical thinking to nursing documentation

FIGURE 7.1 — Eight common charting errors (cont.)

Also ensure that any important health or medication information is documented and communicated to others effectively. Neglecting to communicate an important piece of patient information can leave a nurse open to allegations of negligence. To avoid this, record the information in all of the locations designated by your policies. Also, encourage the use of bright labels and other accepted means of communicating the information.

2. Failure to record nursing actions

There needs to be a way to communicate every nursing action, and nurses must get into the habit of documenting them as close as possible to the time they occur. Unfortunately, charting is often left to the end of many nurses' busy days. This is not a good habit, but often difficult to break. Here are some guidelines to follow:

- Record all observations, assessments, and actions on the flow sheet or designated form.
- You must chart as close to the time as possible, even if it is a one- or two-line entry.
- Reduce redundancy and only chart the fact once. You do not need to repeat the same data in more than one place. Just be sure it can be found in the clinical record. If there is redundancy in your documentation system, revise it.

3. Failure to record medications given

This may seem obvious, but how many times have you reviewed a medication administration record (MAR) and found that the previous shift's nurse said in his or her report that the resident had been medicated even though you could not find it documented in the medical record?

Avoid nursing negligence by recording all medications given and the rationale for those not given, even if you may perceive them as insignificant. Always investigate when you suspect that a medication may have been administered but not recorded.

4. Recording on the wrong chart

Sometimes, a simple mistake of misfiling can lead a nurse to chart on the wrong resident. Staff are especially vulnerable to this error when residents with similar names are on the same unit, so you need a system of identification that is clear and as foolproof as possible.

Chapter 7

> **FIGURE 7.1** — Eight common charting errors (cont.)
>
> Errors in this category include:
> - Transcribing medication orders onto the wrong resident's chart.
> - Writing progress notes without confirming the accuracy of the chart you chose. To prevent this error, look at the external name on the chart and always look at the name stamped at the top of the document.
>
> Whenever possible, do not assign the same nurse to residents with the same name. And always ensure compliance with the National Patient Safety Goal that refers to proper resident identification prior to procedures and medication administration.
>
> **5. Failure to document a discontinued medication**
> Nurses are responsible for ensuring safe resident care at all levels. When a medication has been ordered to be discontinued, the change must be appropriately noted according to policy and communicated to the next shift's nurse. Nurses also need to comply with the organization's policies concerning cross-checking the physician orders with the MAR. Doing so can prevent serious complications.
>
> **6. Failure to document drug reactions/changes in resident's condition**
> The literature on "failure to rescue" points to this potential error. Nurses are responsible for the assessment of a resident's reaction to medication and for the identification of any change in a resident's condition. They must have the skill and knowledge to anticipate the clinical needs of a resident. They must also possess critical-thinking skills to intervene appropriately in any adverse reaction or worsening of the resident's condition. But performing this assessment, identification, and intervention is not enough. Nurses must also document that they have done so.
>
> **7. Improper transcription of orders or transcription of improper orders**
> The registered nurse can be held liable for transcribing improper doses that led to a resident's injury. The nurse can also be held liable for transcribing and carrying out an order they know to be inaccurate or suspect to be incorrect.
>
> If the nurses discuss both the order and their concerns with physicians, they must document these conversations. In addition, if nurses still maintain that administration of the medication or proceeding with a procedure is not in the best interest of the resident, they must activate the chain of command and document that as well.

Applying critical thinking to nursing documentation

> **FIGURE 7.1** Eight common charting errors (cont.)
>
> In contemporary nursing practice, all nurses must know medications or research a new medication prior to administration. If a nurse is not familiar with a procedure and does not seek supervision or assistance with it, questions of clinical competence and ensuring resident safety will come into play if there is any question of malpractice. The public expects that we will continue to keep our professional skills and knowledge up to date. Falling short of this will put a nurse in a difficult position from which to defend him- or herself.
>
> **8. Writing illegible or incomplete records**
> Illegible handwriting is no longer tolerated by regulatory and accreditation surveyors. With the goal of improving resident safety, the days of laughing at someone's handwriting are over. All providers who document in the clinical record must ensure that what they have written is readable. Should the clinical record be reviewed, it is essential that the author of the record be able to clearly read it. Some nursing homes have instituted illegible handwriting policies to improve compliance with legible-documentation standards and to improve resident safety.

Source: DuClos-Miller, P. 2004. *Managing Documentation Risk: A Guide for Nurse Managers.* Marblehead, MA: HCPro, Inc.

Examples of critical writing skills for long-term care nursing

The following are examples of the application of critical writing skills.

Chapter 7

> **Resident case 1**
>
> You are assigned to the skilled unit in a nursing home. Due to a call-out, you are working with only one other RN on the night shift.
>
> **0620 AM**
>
> Physician notified that resident was sent to the Happy Days Hospital via life squad after being found nonresponsive and after initiation of CPR.
>
> **0625 AM**
>
> Family (name and relationship) notified that resident was sent via ambulance to Happy Days Hospital after being found nonresponsive and after receiving CPR.
>
> **0700 AM**
>
> Called Happy Days Hospital to check on resident's status. Resident was admitted to the cardiac intensive care unit with a diagnosis of myocardial infarction.

The documentation shows that the long-term care nurse exhibited autonomy and responsibility. The nurse exhibited independent thinking and actions by calling the code and immediately starting CPR at the same time as moving quickly to support the resident. In a small facility it is important to pull the team together to assist, but also to ensure that other residents' needs are met.

Applying critical thinking to nursing documentation

> **Resident case 2**
>
> The long-term care nurse is caring for Ms. Jones, a 76-year-old Caucasian female admitted for emergent cholecystectomy yesterday. She is postop day 1. The surgeon attempted to remove the gall bladder laparoscopically, but had to resort to an open cholecystectomy due to adhesions and an inability to visualize the gall bladder. Ms. Jones has a T-tube in place that is draining large amounts of bile.
>
> **0800 AM**
>
> Resident dangled for the first time on the side of the bed. Stated she needed to have a bowel movement and ambulated with one-person assist to BR. Pt gait stable and minimal assist needed. States pain 2 out of 10 during ambulation.
>
> **0815 AM**
>
> Ms. Jones found crying inconsolably in the BR. States she is "a freak" and is pointing to the T-tube drainage bag. States that she is a freak because she is "bleeding green blood like Mr. Spock." Calmed and explained to her that it is not blood she is seeing but bile. Assisted back to bed and instruction done re: cholecystectomy and reason for the T-tube being in place temporarily.
>
> **0820 AM**
>
> Ms. Jones visibly calmer and stating, "Now I'm a freak because I freaked out for no reason." Seems embarrassed by her outburst. Pain continues to be 2 out of 10 at this time.

The long-term care nurse uses critical-thinking skills by identifying that the resident needed resident education about the procedure that was done and the resulting additional drainage that was not expected. The nurse is analytical and insightful when questioning the resident about her pain level due to the fact that anxiety is known to increase the perception of pain. The nurse is alert to the context of the situation. The nurse shows empathy by calming the resident and being respectful of the embarrassment the resident feels for her reaction.

Chapter 7

Resident case 3

The nurse is on the medical-surgical unit caring for a resident who is postop 6 hours from a Burch repair. A Foley catheter is intact on a graduated collection device (urometer), IV D51/2NS infusing at 125cc/hour. The resident is taking sips of clear liquids with no nausea or vomiting, and I+O is monitored hourly. The resident received a 500cc bolus in the OR due to low blood pressure. The resident's blood pressure is currently stable.

0920 AM
Called to resident's room for complaint of right flank pain. Resident found in bed doubled over in pain. States pain "an 11" on a scale of 1–10. States pain clearly in flank and not from surgical incision. Noted that resident's urometer was emptied for the hourly assessment by the nursing assistant 20 minutes ago for 15cc of pale yellow urine. Urometer currently contains 5cc pale yellow urine. Catheter tubing traced from point of insertion to collection. No occlusions noted. Review of the chart indicates that pt has been producing approximately 15–20cc per hour since surgery. Unable to palpate bladder. Ultrasound bladder scanner used to identify 10cc urine in bladder. Resident calmed and reassured and pain medication given. Vital signs stable.

0921 AM
Review of chart indicates resident received a total of 1000cc of fluid intraoperatively and has since received a total of 750cc IV fluid and 300cc oral intake. Output has been 120cc over the last 6 hours. No excessive diaphoresis noted. Estimated blood loss during surgery 300cc. No obvious drainage on incisional dressing and no peripheral edema evident. IV flow decreased to TKVO rate. Pt kept NPO as a precaution. Surgeon notified of low urine output.

0923 AM
Right kidney ultrasound ordered. Pt taken to radiology. Pain currently 6 out of 10.

0935 AM
Interdisciplinary note: Radiology – Ultrasound of Rt kidney reveals 1.5 cm hydroureter. Previous films show negative for hydroureter. Discussed with surgeon and decision for exploratory laparascopy identified.

Applying critical thinking to nursing documentation

> **Resident case 3 (cont.)**
>
> **0940 AM**
> Pt returned from radiology with orders to prepare for surgery. Pain continues to increase in spite of medication. Currently reporting 8 out of 10. Surgeon aware and ordered additional medication. Consent obtained prior to administration of medication.
>
> **0950 AM**
> Resident transported to OR via stretcher with surgeon in attendance for exploratory laparascopy for suspected occlusion of R ureter.

The long-term care nurse exhibits critical-thinking skills by collecting the data needed to make an evidence-based assessment. The nurse displays inquisitiveness in finding out if the contusion is clearly in flank and not from surgical incision. Another indication of inquiry is the review of the chart to establish low urine output for an extended period of time although there should be sufficient fluid in the resident's system to have adequate output. The nurse is analytical in establishing that the bladder is not full and that there is no mechanical interruption of the flow through occlusion of the tubing. Further analysis of the overall intake and output to determine fluid balance is another indication of critical thinking and an attempt to problem-solve the situation on behalf of the resident. The nurse displays autonomy in reviewing the chart to collect enough data that the surgeon will take appropriate action to assess the resident further, and is prudent in reducing the IV flow to TKVO rate, and keeping the resident NPO as a precaution.

These examples of documentation of critical thinking in a medical-surgical unit are not unusual. The need for objective recording of information that clearly details the process used by the nurse in assessing, analyzing, evaluating, and taking action for the safety of the resident are the ideal.

Chapter 8
Relating critical thinking to its higher purpose

By Polly Gerber Zimmermann, RN, MS, MBA, CEN

In nursing, we tend to work toward achieving goals as the end of a process, when many times meeting the goal is just the beginning. In this book, Polly Gerber Zimmermann reminds us that learning to think critically is a journey, not a destination. The foundation of critical-thinking skills you build for nurses will be directly reflected in your ability to continue on this path. The ability to meet the needs of our residents is a moving walkway that seems to go on forever. Each specialty of healthcare delivery is faced with having to provide care to more residents at a faster pace with fewer resources.

Whether you work in skilled nursing, assisted living, or in any other environment, nurses are the people residents and families turn to. They turn to us for clarification, guidance, hope, and the truth.

> **Critical thinking in every-day life**
>
> While driving home from the hospital, I was listening to a postal worker in New Orleans being interviewed on public radio. The postal worker was delivering mail to a district recently reopened after Hurricane Katrina. The interview went along these lines:
>
> **Q: What kind of challenges are you facing with this delivery area?**
> **A:** Well, there are lots of challenges, such as the debris and trash.
>
> **Q: Is it difficult to tell whether or not it is the right house you are delivering to?**
> **A:** If the number is no longer there or the mailbox is gone, we are supposed to use deductive reasoning to determine if it is the right house. For example, I might look to see if it is a consecutive number.

Chapter 8

This interview reminds us that we use critical thinking in our daily lives without realizing it. For example we think critically:

- At the grocery store to determine if the sale price is really a sale or just a cheaper price on a smaller container

- When our child tells us, "I did study for that exam," yet you never saw a book in his or her room

- At the dentist's, office when we decide whether to pay to fix the tooth or have it pulled

We cannot continue to improve the quality of care we deliver without engaging our reasoning. The ability to reason and consider actions or inactions is a feature of critical thinking that provides a safe resident-care environment. Recognizing the best interest of the resident is paramount in quality-improvement processes. As you consider all of the efforts in which your organization is engaged regarding meeting regulatory standards remember this:

Staff members cannot meet the needs of residents if they cannot recognize those needs.

Chapter 9
Resources and tools

By Polly Gerber Zimmermann, RN, MS, MBA, CEN

This chapter contains additional tools and resources to assist you in assessing and developing medical-surgical nurses' critical-thinking capabilities at the point of hire, during orientation, and through ongoing development and review. This chapter contains:

- A list of further reading and resources

- Additional sample questions

- Figure 9.1, which is a handout that can be given to attendees of a critical-thinking class who want further information and study materials

- Figure 9.2, which contains unfolding teaching scenarios that can be used for discussing critical thinking

- Figure 9.3, which contains examples of teachable moments

- Figure 9.4, which is a teaching tool about critical thinking and skills related to geriatric residents

- Figure 9.5, which is a sample critical-thinking-skills class agenda that can be customized for any facility

- Figures 9.6–9.11 are worksheets that can be used or adapted for critical-thinking classes, during orientation, or for ongoing critical-thinking development.

Resources and further reading

Publications

Alfaro-Lefevre, R. 2004. *Critical Thinking and Clinical Judgment: A Practical Approach*. St. Louis: WB Saunders.

Chapter 9

Black, J. M., Hawks, J. H., and Keene, A.M. 2004. *Medical-Surgical Nursing: Clinical Management for Positive Outcomes*. Philadelphia: WB Saunders.

Doan-Johnson, S., and A. Woods, eds. 2005. *Nursing Made Incredibly Easy*. Philadelphia: Lippincott Williams & Wilkins.

DuClos-Miller, P. 2004. *Managing Documentation Risk: A Guide for Nurse Managers*. Marblehead, MA: HCPro, Inc.

Goodman, B. 2006. "How to ask an intelligent question." *Nursing Standard* 20 (24): 81.

Hsu, L., and S. Hsieh. 2005. "Concept maps as an assessment tool in a nursing course." *Journal of Professional Nursing* 21 (3): 141–149.

Ignatavicius, D. D., and M. L. Workman. 2006. *Medical-Surgical Nursing: Critical Thinking for Collaborative Care*, 2-Volume Set. Philadelphia: Elsevier Saunders.

Lauri, S.; Salantera, S.; Chalmers, K.; Ekmann, S.; Hesook, S.; Kappeli, S.; and MacLeod, M. 2001. "An exploratory study of clinical decision-making in five countries." *Journal of Nursing Scholarship* 33 (1): 83–90.

Lipe, S. K.; and Beasley, S. 2004. *Critical Thinking in Nursing: A Cognitive Skills Workbook*. Philadelphia: Lippincott Williams & Wilkins.

Myrick, F., and Yonge, O. 2002. "Preceptor questioning and student thinking." *Journal of Professional Nursing* 18 (3): 176–181.

Profetto-McGrath, J. 2005. "Critical thinking and evidence-based practice." *Journal of Professional Nursing* 21 (6): 364–371.

Rubenfeld, M. G., and Scheffer, B. K. 2006. *Critical Thinking Tactics for Nurses*. Sudbury, MA: Jones and Bartlett.

Scheffer, B. K. 2006. "Critical thinking: A tool in search of a job." *Journal of Nursing Education* 45 (6): 195–196.

Springhouse. 2003. *Medical-Surgical Nursing Made Incredibly Easy!* Philadelphia: Lippincott Williams & Wilkins.

Springhouse. 2004. *Fluids and Electrolytes Made Incredibly Easy!* Philadelphia: Lippincott Williams & Wilkins.

Springhouse. 2004. *Nurses Legal Handbook.* Philadelphia: Lippincott Williams & Wilkins.

Springhouse. 2006. *Professional Guide to Signs & Symptoms*, 5th ed. Philadelphia: Lippincott Williams & Wilkins.

Tanner, C. A. 2006. "Thinking like a nurse: A research-based model of clinical judgment in nursing." *Journal of Nursing Education* 45 (6): 204–211.

Thompson, C. 2001. "Clinical decision making in nursing: Theoretical perspectives and their relevance to practice—a response to Jean Harbison." *Journal of Advanced Nursing* 35 (1): 134–137.

Wright, D. 2005. *The Ultimate Guide to Competency Assessment in Healthcare.* Eau Claire, WI: PFSI Healthcare.

Yocum, F. 1999. *Documentation Skills for Quality Patient Care.* Dayton, OH: Awareness Productions.

Web sites

Enchanted Learning: *www.enchantedlearning.com*

- Anatomy diagrams/glossaries and more

North Central Regional Educational Laboratory (NCREL®): *www.ncrel.org*

- Resources defining critical thinking

Chapter 9

The Advisory Board Company: *www.advisory.com*

- Multiple resources: Search under new graduate nurse

National Council of State Boards of Nursing: *www.ncsbn.org*

- Access to all State Boards of Nursing rules and regulations

The Institute for Family-Centered Care: *www.familycenteredcare.org*

- Promotes collaboration between care provider and family, offering educational material and other professional resources for family-centered care at home and in the hospital

Healthy People 2010: *www.HealthyPeople.gov*

- Federally funded series of national health objectives that aims to identify preventable threats to health and set goals to reduce them; look for professional resources including sections on the Best Practice Initiative, Implementations, and Leading Health Indicators

American Nurses Association: *www.NursingWorld.org*

- Information on many issues facing the professional nurse today

American Academy of Nurse Practitioners: *www.AANP.org*

- Resource for nurse practitioners to promote excellence in practice, education, and research

Foundation for Critical Thinking: *www.criticalthinking.org*

- Nonprofit organization that works to promote educational reform and promote critical thinking; nonhealthcare-specific

Additional sample questions

Source: Janie Krechting, RN-C, BSN, MGS, LNHA

These questions may be used either for discussion or for a test. Remove answers before providing them to learners. (File can be found under "Additional sample questions" on the accompanying CD-ROM.)

Question: The charge nurse enters the room to give the resident medication. The resident complains of being short of breath.

The best initial action by the nurse is to:

    a. Get the supervisor

    b. Assess the resident

    c. Call the life squad

    d. Call the physician

Answer: B

The nurse will need to get the resident's vital signs, listen to the resident's lung sounds, and get the PO2 level via pulse oximeter. There should be baseline information available prior to notifying the physician.

Question: A 92-year-old female resident has been admitted from the medical-surgical unit to a long-term care facility with a fractured left hip. She has a medical diagnosis of dementia. She appears untidy, suspicious, belligerent, easily antagonized, and her speech is nonsensical. Which of the following should be included in her plan of care?

    a. A speech therapy consult

    b. Pet and/or music therapy referral

    c. Reducing stimuli as much as possible

    d. Only allowing visits from family members she can identify

Answer: B

Chapter 9

After the immediate care needs have occurred—pain management, medication management, and therapy—the priority should be to reduce the symptoms of the dementia as much as possible. This will also assist with pain management. Research has shown that pets and/or music can reduce the impact of changes to place and trauma on those who suffer from dementia.

Response A is inappropriate due to the dementia. Response C is inappropriate due to the fact that residents with dementia will deteriorate further if left alone.

Response D is inappropriate due to the fact that she may not be able to recognize any family. Visitors are, however, an important part of maintaining function in dementia sufferers, along with touch and tactile stimulation.

Question: A resident is admitted with an acute exacerbation of congestive heart failure (CHF). Vital signs are as follows: T 98.9, P 120, R 30, BP 160/98. Peripheral edema is evident to the ankles with +3 pitting edema to mid-calf. Lung sounds reveal crackles to the mid-lobe bilaterally. The provider orders 0.5 mg digoxin and 80 mg furosemide IV push now. Which of the following assessment findings would indicate that the medications are having the desired effect?

    a. Lungs clear to auscultation
    b. Urine-specific gravity increased
    c. Heart rate decrease below 90
    d. Respiratory rate unchanged but deeper intake

Answer: A

The medications are intended to both increase the effectiveness of the cardiac contraction and reduce excess fluid. This is evident in response A.

Response B is incorrect due to the fact that the specific gravity would actually decrease if the excess fluid were being excreted. Response C is partially correct, as the digoxin would decrease the heart rate, but this alone is not sufficient as an assessment that the cardiac effectiveness is improved.

Response D is incorrect as the ease of breathing will be increased, therefore the rate of respiration should be decreased as well. Increased depth of respiration is an indicator of collected CO2 and reveals a different diagnosis than the CHF.

Resources and tools

Question: An 83-year-old female resident was on Lasix, but it was discontinued because the resident's BUN and creatine indicated that the Lasix could contribute to kidney damage. The resident received Aldactone, but did not have additional lab work. The resident began to complain of shortness of breath and chest pain.

Which of the following lab tests is indicated and why?

a. T3
b. T4
c. Potassium
d. INR

Answer: C

Because Aldactone is a potassium-sparing drug, a potassium level would be indicated.

Source for the following questions: Polly Gerber Zimmermann, RN, MS, MBA, CEN

Question: The night nurse walks in to find the resident lying motionless on the floor. List the order in which the nurse should complete the following actions.
(Note: This is the new-style sequential NCLEX question. No partial credit is allowed.)

a. Call the doctor
b. Write an incident report
c. Ask the resident what hurts
d. Place the resident in the bed
e. Ask the resident why he or she got up
f. Assess the pulse

Answer: F, C, D, E, A, B

First, establish whether the resident is conscious. Is this syncope from a dysrhythmia? Then establish whether the resident hit his or her head; rule out neck injury and need for immobilization. Review procedure if that was the case. Could institute a discussion about what resident medications would increase the nurse's concern (warfarin/Coumadin). Then move the resident.

Discuss how often we see people ask E first, but does it really matter? After immediate needs, ask: What is a common reason for falling? Going to the bathroom.

Critical Thinking in Long-Term Care Nursing

Chapter 9

Question: A 96-year-old resident who was admitted with pneumonia is found crawling out of the bed. What should the nurse do first?

    a. Assess the resident's pain level

    b. Obtain a pulse oximeter reading

    c. Reorient the resident and reinforce the need to stay in bed

    d. Apply a Posey jacket

Answer: B

New-onset confusion should have hypoglycemia and inadequate oxygenation ruled out first. The elderly who have decreased respiratory reserve are more prone to complications and atypical presentations.

Follow-up discussion could include how you would handle a low reading, and what else to consider if it was "normal." (How would you expect the result to be different if the resident had COPD?)

One of the most common symptoms for urinary tract infection in residents with Alzheimer's disease is new-onset restlessness.

Could also have a discussion about other considerations: sundowning, alternatives to restraints, etc.

Consider offering a true "war story" as an accompaniment: Resident kept crawling out of bed. Nurse obtained order and restrained resident. Other nurse took pulse oximetry and found it was 88%.

Use this as a good opportunity to review the nursing home's restraint policy.

Question: The nurse receives the following lab values on the newly admitted resident. Which value should the nurse deal with first?
(Note: This is the new-style fill-in-the blank NCLEX question.)
(Note: AST and ALT were formerly known as SGOT and SGPT.)

Test	Resident result	Normal range
Glucose	193 mg/dL	70–110 mg/dL
BUN	8 mg/dL	10–20 mg/dL
Cr	0.7 mg/dL	0.7–1.2 mg/dL
Sodium	131 mEq/dL	136–145 mEq/dL
Potassium	3.2 mEq/dL	3.5–5.0 mEq/dL
SGOT/ALT	1932 IU/L	13–40 IU/L
SGPT/AST	2360 IU/L	7–60 IU/L

Answer: Potassium

Resources and tools

Potassium is an intracellular electrolyte and a drop of 0.1 mEq actually represents a drop of 200 mEq. Since potassium affects muscle, the nurse would be most worried about the effect on cardiac muscle.

Sodium is an extracellular electrolyte, so the results are an actual reflection of the current body supply. In addition, the kidney can conserve sodium, but not potassium.

The elevated glucose could be, in part, due to the acute illness. A further workup or insulin could be done later.

The resident does have liver enzyme elevation but that is not the priority. It would be a factor in drug dosing.

How will this resident appear? Jaundiced.

Question: The nurse receives the following laboratory results for a resident. What is the best interpretation?

Test	Resident result	Normal range
WBC	4.1 K/cmm	4.5–10.0 K/cmm
RBC	3.2 mil/cmm	4.3–5.8 mil/cmm
HGB	11.3 gm/dL	12–15 gm/dL
HCT	29.1%	36–47%
Segs	28%	36–71%
Bands	2%	0–7%
Lymphs	62%	20–40%
Eosinophils	3%	1–6%

a. The resident is immunosuppressed
b. The resident is having an allergic reaction
c. The resident has an acute bacterial infection
d. The resident has a viral infection

Answer: D

Critical Thinking in Long-Term Care Nursing

Chapter 9

Lymphs go up in a viral infection. Depressed, rather than elevated, WBC are more likely with viral. Immunosuppression would result in significant depression of all views. The borderline hemoglobin can also be a result of this. Eosinophils are elevated in an allergic reaction. An acute bacterial infection would typically have an elevated WBC and neutrophils, bands/segs/immature cells.

Question: It is most important for the nurse to care for which new resident complaint first?

    a. Type II DM with a.m. blood sugar of 160 mg
    b. Client receiving a K+ rider (IVPB) complaining that the arm is sore
    c. Asthmatic on steroids is catching the flu, temperature 100.4°F (38°C)
    d. Resident with pneumonia's WBC is 15,000 with an elevation in neutrophils

Answer: C

Rule out septic response in an immunosuppressed resident with compromised respiratory function. Then A can be taken care of.

B is an expected complaint. What can the nurse do? It might be possible to slow the infusion rate or further dilute the concentration.

D is an expected finding. What else does the nurse want to know? Resident's temperature and the trend of the WBC: higher, lower, the same. Also verify the resident is on an appropriate antibiotic.

Resources and tools

FIGURE 9.1 — Critical thinking skills course—Additional resources handout

- **Dorothy Del Bueno's article about critical thinking displayed by nurses:** Del Bueno, D. 2001. "Buyer beware: The cost of competence." *Nursing Economics* 19 (6): 257–259.

- **American Association of Critical-Care Nursing (AACN) decision tree for delegation decisions:** Available from 101 Columbia, Alisa Viejo, CA 92656-1491; 800/899-2226.

- **Give new graduates "rules" for "telling somebody" by using the criteria developed for Rapid Response Team Activation** (a concept introduced by the Institute for Healthcare Improvement [IHI] as part of the "100,000 Lives Campaign.")

- IHI recommendations: *www.ihi.org/IHI/Programs/TransformingCareattheBedside*.

- Scholle, C. C., and C. Mininni. 2006. "Best-practice interventions: How a Rapid Response Team saves lives." *Nursing2006* 36 (1): 36–40.
    - Mean arterial pressure < 70 or > 130 mmHg
    - Heart rate < 45 or > 125
    - Respiratory rate < 10 or > 30
    - Complaints of chest pain
    - Change in mental status (lasting more than 10 minutes)

According to one study, 66% of patients had signs of instability for up to eight hours prior to the event. Studies have shown that up to 70% of the calls to a Rapid Response Team were based on concerns about the patient's respiratory status, accompanied by staff concern about a patient's deteriorating condition.

"Brains in our Pocket" resources for nurses
- PDA programs:
    - See Audrey Snyder's chapter "PDA Use" in P. G. Zimmermann and R. D. Herr, 2006, *Triage Nursing Secrets* (St. Louis: Mosby/Elsevier) for suggested programs and sources to obtain them.

Chapter 9

> **FIGURE 9.1** Critical thinking skills course—Additional resources handout (cont.)
>
> - Print:
>   - Myers, E. 2003. *RNotes: Nurse's Clinical Pocket Guide*. Philadelphia: FA Davis.
>
> **Good sources of test questions**
> - LaCharity, L. A., C. D. Kumagai, and B. Bartz. 2005. *Prioritization, Delegation & Assignment Practice Exercises for Medical-Surgical Nursing*. St. Louis: Mosby/Elsevier.
> - Springhouse. 2006. *NCLEX-RN: 250 New-Format Questions*. Philadelphia: Lippincott Williams & Wilkins.
> - Rayfield, S., and L. Manning. 2004. *NCLEX-RN 101: How to Pass!*, 5th ed. Gulf Shores, AL: ICAN.
>
> **Aids for writing better test questions**
> - Bosher, S. 2003. "Linguistic bias in multiple-choice nursing exams." *Nursing Education Perspectives* 24 (1): 25–34.
> - Zimmermann, P. G. 2005. "Writing effective test questions." *Journal of Emergency Nursing* 32 (1): 106–109.
>
> **Concept mapping**
> - Carpenito-Moyet, L. J. 2005. *Understanding the Nursing Process: Concept Mapping and Care Planning for Students*. Philadelphia: Lippincott Williams & Wilkins.
> - Schuster, P. M. 2000. "Concept mapping: Reducing clinical care plan paperwork and increasing learning." *Nurse Educator* 25 (2): 76–81.
>
> **Critical-thinking books**
> - Rubenfeld, M. G., and B. K. Scheffer. 2006. *Critical Thinking Tactics for Nurses*. Sudbury, MA: Jones and Bartlett.
> - Lipe, S. K., and S. Beasley. 2004. *Critical Thinking in Nursing: A Cognitive Skills Workbook*. Philadelphia: Lippincott Williams & Wilkins.

| FIGURE 9.1 | Critical thinking skills course—Additional resources handout (cont.) |

Generation X/multigenerational work force
- Duchscher, J. E. B., and L. Cowin. 2004. "Multigenerational nurses in the workplace." *Journal of Nursing Administration* 34 (11): 493–501.
- Lower, J. 2006. *A Practical Guide to Managing the Multigenerational Workforce: Skills for Nurse Managers*. Marblehead, MA: HCPro.
- Raines, C. 2002. "Managing Generation X Employees" in P. G. Zimmermann's *Nursing Management Secrets*. Philadelphia: Hanley & Belfus.
- Raines, C. 1997. *Beyond Generation X*. Menlo Park, CA: Crisp.
- Sacks, P. 1996. *Generation X Goes to College*. Chicago and LaSalle, IL: Open Court.

Example of a worst-case scenario
- Zimmermann, P. G. (2003) "Lessons learned: On watching for zebras." *Journal of Emergency Nursing* 29 (1): 85–86.

Source: Polly Gerber Zimmermann, RN, MS, MBA, CEN

Chapter 9

> **FIGURE 9.2** Unfolding teaching scenarios for long-term care nurses
>
> These scenarios can be used as discussion areas during critical-thinking classes or adapted and given to nurses for further reading.
>
> ## Scenario 1
>
> ### Who-When-What-Think-Ask-Do
>
> **Who:** 20-year-old female
> **When:** Postoperative day 1, laparascopic appendectomy
> **What:** Patient states that she is having lower abdominal pain across the entire lower abdomen, and up into the epigastric area as well.
>
> ### New graduate nurse thinks:
> "Oh no, possible peritonitis due to rupture of the appendix."
>
> ### REMEMBER
> When you hear hoof beats in a patient, first look for horses, not zebras.
>
> **Think:** The patient was assessed intraoperatively for any signs of rupture of the appendix before it was removed. There was no indication of rupture in the operative report.
>
> **Ask:** Does the pain move based on patient position? Yes.
> Is the patient passing flatus? Yes.
> Is the patient taking and tolerating PO fluids? Yes.
>
> **Do:** Observe/Assess:
> Any rebound tenderness across the abdomen? No.
> Surgery was done using laparascopic equipment? Yes.
> Any excessive bleeding from operative sites? No.
> Any obvious distention of abdomen as compared to first assessment? No.
> Patient voiding quantity sufficient (QS) amounts? Yes.
>
> ### Diagnose:
> Pain related to excess carbon dioxide in abdomen post-laparascopic procedure

| FIGURE 9.2 | Unfolding teaching scenarios for long-term care nurses (cont.) |

Intervene:
- Educate patient regarding the process used to inflate the abdomen for increased visibility during the procedure
- Identify the common side effects of CO2 use
- Encourage movement to facilitate blood flow to the peritoneum and absorption of the excess CO2
- Provide nonnarcotic pain medication to alleviate pain, and reassess for need for narcotic if not effective

Scenario 2

Who-When-What-Think-Ask-Do

Who: The emergency department calls to report that a 94-year-old female with suspected hip fracture, unknown to your facility, is en route to the hospital via ambulance and will be admitted directly to the unit for treatment. The orthopedic surgeon is en route.

When the patient arrives you are given a report by the emergency medical technicians.

When: The patient speaks no English. Her language and dress indicate that she is from somewhere in the Middle East. Her husband is at her side and will not leave her. He is significantly younger than she is and appears to be in his late 60s. Her left leg is contracted and shorter than the right and she is thrashing on the stretcher due to pain.

What: You prepare to perform a full admission physical examination, but when you lift the blanket you realize that the patient has been physically abused for a prolonged period of time as you note numerous bruises in various stages of resolution. You note the husband is staring at you.

What is your first action?

REMEMBER
Think before acting. Respond to the situation, don't react to it.

Chapter 9

> **FIGURE 9.2** Unfolding teaching scenarios for long-term care nurses (cont.)
>
> **Think:** What do I need to do to provide this woman, and her husband, safe and effective care?
>
> **Ask:** Can I provide this patient and her husband with the best care possible while putting my feelings about abuse of the elderly aside?
>
> **Do:** Because you cannot assume that it was the husband that abused her you need to proceed with the physical examination and note the presence of the bruises.
> Ask the husband if he has seen the bruises before and what the explanation of them may be.
> Report your findings to the surgeon and request a social work consult for a home/caregiver assessment.
>
> **INSTRUCTOR:**
> - Prompt students to think why these specific actions are important
> - If no response, prompt application of knowledge of abuse and how the knowledge of the home situation could be applied to the elderly
> - Guide the students through the steps, associating the possible ramifications of bringing the abuse to public scrutiny in this culture versus the patient's original cultural environment
> - Discuss transcultural nursing and transcultural caring
>
> ## Scenario 3
>
> ### *Who-When-What-Think-Ask-Do*
>
> **Who, When, What:** You are an intermittent nurse in the medical-surgical float pool. The surgical gynecology/urology unit of your hospital has had an overwhelming number of admissions in the past 24 hours and you are assigned there for this shift.
>
> **Your assignment is as follows:**
> **Patient 1:** Mrs. A
> 25 years old
> Postoperative two hours from D&C for incomplete abortion
> Moderate amount of sanguinous flow
> VS stable

FIGURE 9.2	**Unfolding teaching scenarios for long-term care nurses (cont.)**

Patient 2: Mr. B

24 years old

Receiving IV antibiotics for treatment of gonorrhea

Newly diagnosed HIV positive

Follow-up needed re: sexual partners and education about the transmission of HIV

Patient 3: Mr. C

54 years old

One day postoperative of a radical retropubic prostatectomy

Ambulating with two-person assist, IV fluids, Foley catheter, hemovac drains

Wife teary due to surgeon's statement that they could not preserve the nerves

Patient 4: Mrs. D

34 years old

Postoperative day 1, bilateral mastectomy for breast cancer

Local news anchorwoman

Difficulty controlling visitors

Patient 5: Ms. E

19 years old

Acute renal colic

History of cocaine and heroin abuse

Patient arguing and shouting throughout the day due to lack of pain management

Security called X2 to control visitors

After receiving report you feel overwhelmed and think this assignment may be more than you can handle since you are called to this unit so infrequently. You also realize that the unit nurses are carrying even heavier patient loads due to the increased census and short staff situation.

What do you do?

Chapter 9

> **FIGURE 9.2** Unfolding teaching scenarios for long-term care nurses (cont.)

INSTRUCTOR:
- Ask students for possible actions this nurse can take
- Discuss the ethics of this situation with the students
- Relate this situation to "knowing what you don't know"

REMEMBER
Fear of the unknown can rob you of your power.

Think: What does my assignment actually entail? Break it down and put it in perspective.

Ask: Now that the assignment is put into perspective, does it still look unmanageable? Reassess.

- Do I feel comfortable with this assignment?
- If I still don't feel comfortable with the assignment, do I have any options? What exactly are those options?
- Am I willing to exercise those options with the potential for appearing to be less of a "team player" to my peers?
- Is there anything unethical or illegal about any of my options?
- Will I accept the assignment even if it appears to be more than I can handle safely?

Do: Take action on your decision.

- What are the possible actions you could take?
  - Accept assignment
  - Refuse assignment
  - Accept assignment under duress
  - Ask for a different assignment
  - Share assignment with a regular staff member on that unit

Resources and tools

FIGURE 9.3 — Skilled unit teachable moments

Case 1

Who-When-What-Think-Ask-Do

Who, when, what: You are assigned to the day shift and are caring for a patient who had an acute exacerbation of his congestive heart failure due to eating foods high in sodium and not taking the prescribed antihypertensive medications. The patient received IV Lasix, has been stabilized on his antihypertensive medications, and is being discharged to home with his wife. You have been given report that discharge teaching was provided during the night shift. You have read the night shift nurse's notes that state she gave discharge instructions to both the patient and his wife.

Think: What is your next course of action?

Ask: Am I able to document that I discharged this family to home with full discharge instructions and am I sure that they know how to care for this chronic illness?

REMEMBER

When in doubt about a course of action to be taken, think about what questions would be asked of you, and how you would answer them, if they were being asked by an attorney or an ethicist.

Do: Ask questions that reveal the patient's level of understanding of the discharge teaching:
- Is the patient able to describe the actions he took that lead to him being admitted to the hospital this time?
- Do the patient and his wife have a written instruction sheet including the phone number of a contact person they should call to report an increase in edema, shortness of breath, heartbeat irregularities, or to ask further questions?
- Do the patient and his wife know WHEN and for WHAT situations to call the contact person?
- If presented with a hypothetical scenario do the patient and his wife respond with the appropriate action to be taken for the situation?

Chapter 9

> **FIGURE 9.3** — Skilled unit teachable moments (cont.)
>
> Document that you are discharging this family home and your assurance that they are capable of caring for this patient and his chronic illness.
>
> ### REMEMBER
> Even though discharge instructions were given on night shift, you are the nurse who is releasing this family from the care of the hospital.
>
> ## Case 2
>
> ### Who-When-What-Think-Ask-Do
>
> **Who, when, what:** You are the preceptor of a new orientee who is working your assignment for the shift with you. As you check the crash carts in your area you notice items are missing and some medications are out of date. There was a new system put in place to catch issues such as this so it is surprising to see that this has happened.
>
> **Think:** The nurse recognizes that the system may have a break in it that needs to be addressed.
>
> **Ask:** How should I manage the system issue?
> Can the orientee verbalize how noncompliance with the system can affect care?
> Can the orientee identify where and how to obtain a new crash cart and where to return this one for restocking?
> Does the orientee understand what paperwork needs to be filled out?
>
> **Do:** The nurse notifies the central supply department and pharmacy that the cart was inappropriately stocked and shows the orientee how to process the paperwork required.

FIGURE 9.3 — Skilled unit teachable moments (cont.)

Case 3

Who-When-What-Think-Ask-Do

Who, when, what: Your orientee approaches you to share that yesterday the nurse she was shadowing had a patient with blunt trauma to the abdomen. The orientee was surprised that the nurse spent a tremendous amount of time focused on placing an NG tube. She was surprised by this especially since the patient's blood pressure kept dropping.

Think: The nurse is able to identify the physiology and implications of abdominal bleeding.

Ask: The nurse should ask how to prioritize care. Ask the orientee how care should have been prioritized if not the way the nurse preceptor was prioritizing.
Identify why the BP was dropping.
What impact would constant vomiting have on the airway?
How did the orientee approach the nurse preceptor when she felt the priorities were out of order?

Do: The nurse reviews the anatomy and pathophysiology, lab values, physician orders, and the teaching plan, noting any special needs of the patient.

Chapter 9

| FIGURE 9.4 | Critical-thinking skills and the frail elderly in the nursing home setting |

Critical thinking requires knowledge, experience, and the ability to judge what is in the best interest of the resident.

- Be curious about things
- Ask pertinent questions
- Examine problems closely before assuming anything
- Seek resources and advice when you don't understand
- Reject advice that says, "That's the way we've always done it around here"
- Be open-minded
- Identify incorrect information and reject it

1. 78-year-old male resident with a history of arthritis.

Resident states: *"The medicine doesn't work. I don't feel any better. I feel weak."* Pulse is 110.

- What question will you respond with to the resident?
- How can you clarify the resident's expectations of the medicine?
- What medication complication could be present?
- Is there really a medical problem, or is this an issue of lack of communication?

2. 67-year-old female resident with a history of hypertension presents with blood pressure of 176/112.

Resident states: *"I feel just fine. I don't know what all the fuss is about."*

- What question will you respond with to the resident?
- Can you clarify the resident's perception of what her diagnosis of hypertension means?
- Do you need to verify compliance with medical treatment since she claims to feel fine?

| FIGURE 9.4 | Critical thinking skills and the frail elderly in the nursing home setting (cont.) |

3. 92-year-old male has been examined by the provider. You are about to change his dressing.

Resident states: *"The doctor just told me everything is okay. But I know something is wrong they are not telling me about."* He is now crying and appears anxious.

- What question will you respond with to the resident?
- Other than his medical condition, what might his emotions be related to?

Source: Shelley Cohen, RN, BS, CEN, and Janie Krechting RN-C, BSN, MGS, LNHA

Chapter 9

FIGURE 9.5 — Sample agenda

[Your facility]
Critical-Thinking Skills
[Date of program]

9:00–9:15	**Introduction to critical thinking and course overview**
9:15–10:00	**Resident assessments**
	MDS explanation
	Risk assessment explanation
	Fall risk, pressure ulcer risk, elopement risk
	Establishing the baseline
	Reassessments
10:00–10:15	**Stretch break**
10:15–11:30	**Frail elderly resident**
	Polypharmacy issues
	Atypical presentations
	Abuse protocols and reporting
11:30–12:15	**Lunch**
12:15–1:15	**Red flags**
	Resident statements/comments
	Family input and care conferences
	Documentation specifics
	Case scenarios
1:15–1:30	**Stretch break**
1:30–2:30	**Applying the knowledge**
	When to call the doctor
	More case scenarios
2:30	**Course evaluations**

Source: Shelley Cohen, RN, BS, CEN, and Janie Krechting RN-C, BSN, MGS, LNHA

Resources and tools

FIGURE 9.6 — Instructor worksheet—Connecting words to spark critical thinking

In each of these resident cases, what question(s) should you consider?

(Instructor notes contain what to ask or what you want the nurse to consider.)

1. Resident states she has no pain relief after the medication you gave her.

(Instructor note: Why is there no pain relief?)

2. A 95-year-old female resident with blood pressure of 180/95 sustained even after medication administered.

(Instructor note: Any other signs and symptoms of note? What questions should you ask the resident?)

3. When changing the dressing of a resident with a stage IV pressure ulcer, you notice green, foul-smelling drainage.

(Instructor note: What time was the last dressing change noted in the chart? What has happened to cause the change in the wound? Has the MD been notified? Is the resident on antibiotics? Are there other signs or symptoms of infection? Is the resident septic?

4. Resident who had a fall and hit head has had a change in his level of consciousness.

(Instructor note: Further assessment of wound drainage should include what area and why? Who noted the change? Staff, family? What examples are offered as to evidence of the change? Are the vital signs stable? Does the resident with a head injury have increased intracranial pressure? Should the resident be sent to the hospital? Have the MD and family been notified?

Source: Shelley Cohen, RN, BS, CEN, and June Marshall, RN, MS, CNAA, BC

Chapter 9

> **FIGURE 9.7** Nurse worksheet—Connecting words to spark critical thinking
>
> Following each of these resident statements, what question(s) should you consider?
>
> 1. Resident states she has no pain relief after the medication you gave her.
>
> 2. A 95-year-old female resident with blood pressure of 180/95 sustained even after medication administered.
>
> 3. When changing the dressing of a resident with a stage IV pressure ulcer, you notice green, foul-smelling drainage.
>
> 4. Resident who had a fall and hit head has had a change in his level of consciousness.

Source: Shelley Cohen, RN, BS, CEN; Kelly A. Goudreau, DSN, RN, CNS-BC; and Janie Krechting RN-C, BSN, MGS, LNHA

FIGURE 9.8	Worksheet—Relationship to critical thinking

How do each of these items below relate to critical thinking? Give one resident example for each.

Invasive therapy/treatment/indwelling devices
- Intravenous
- Catheters/devices
- Tubes
  - Nasogastric
  - Suprapubic
  - Feeding
- Colostomy
- Urostomy
- Dressings
- Wounds
- Orthopedic devices

Chapter 9

| FIGURE 9.9 | Worksheet—Vital signs |

In each set of resident vital signs below, what question would you ask the resident? What other areas would you assess?

Vital signs + Assessment = Critical thinking

"A critical thinker is able to reject information that is incorrect or irrelevant."
—S. Ferrett

Case 1
Temp	97.4 (rectal)
Pulse	118
Respirations	26
Blood Pressure	128/72

Case 2
Temp	95.5 (po)
Pulse	62
Respirations	30
Blood Pressure	192/66

Case 3
Temp	102.4
Pulse	78
Respirations	14
Blood Pressure	78/52

Source: Shelley Cohen, RN, BS, CEN

Resources and tools

FIGURE 9.10 Worksheet—Red-flag alerts

Resident statement/question	Makes you think . . .	Your response is . . .
I haven't had a bowel movement in a week		
My stool has been black and tarry, and I feel weak and dizzy		
Since I fell and hit my head last week when getting up to go to the bathroom, I have been having headaches and vomiting		
Since I started on the new medication, my tongue has been protruding and my hands have been shaking		
I keep feeling dizzy when I stand up		
I feel really thirsty; my tongue is dry and my eyes look sunken and red around the periphery		
I have a new sore on my bottom since I came here		
That nursing assistant yelled at me		

Source: Shelley Cohen, RN, BS, CEN; Kelly A. Goudreau, DSN, RN, CNS-BC; and Janie Krechting, RN-C, BSN, MGS, LNHA

Chapter 9

> **FIGURE 9.11** — Worksheet—Relating nursing care to critical thinking
>
> For each of the following skills, procedures, or interventions, answer the questions below:
> - IV access/therapy
> - Cardiac/respiratory monitoring
> - Enteral feeding via gastric tube
> - Nasopharyngeal/oropharyngeal suctioning
> - Pain assessment and management
> - Medical immobilization (use of restraints)
> - Reporting suspected abuse or neglect
>
> 1. Why would the resident need this?
>
> 2. What is my role in this?
>
> 3. How will I know it's safe?
>
> 4. Will I be able to adequately assess the efficacy of this procedure/intervention?
>
> 5. What are the risks/benefits of this?
>
> 6. What observations/considerations should I make in regard to this intervention?
>
> 7. Does the resident have any cultural/ethnic beliefs or practices that will have an effect on this procedure/intervention?
>
> 8. Will this procedure/intervention impact negatively on the intra/interfamily privacy issues?

Source: Shelley Cohen, RN, BS, CEN; Kelly A. Goudreau, DSN, RN, CNS-BC; and Janie Krechting RN-C, BSN, MGS, LNHA